MANAGING MIGRAINE
IN PRIMARY CARE

Managing Migraine in Primary Care

ANNE MACGREGOR

Blackwell
Science

© 1999 by
Blackwell Science Ltd
Editorial Offices:
Osney Mead, Oxford OX2 0EL
25 John Street, London WC1N 2BL
23 Ainslie Place, Edinburgh EH3 6AJ
350 Main Street, Malden
  MA 02148 5018, USA
54 University Street, Carlton
  Victoria 3053, Australia
10, rue Casimir Delavigne
  75006 Paris, France

Other Editorial Offices:
Blackwell Wissenschafts-Verlag GmbH
Kurfürstendamm 57
10707 Berlin, Germany

Blackwell Science KK
MG Kodenmacho Building
7–10 Kodenmacho Nihombashi
Chuo-ku, Tokyo 104, Japan

The right of the Author to be
identified as the Author of this Work
has been asserted in accordance
with the Copyright, Designs and
Patents Act 1988.

First published 1999

Set by Sparks Computer Solutions, Oxford
Printed and bound in Great Britain at the
Alden Press, Oxford and Northampton

The Blackwell Science logo is a
trade mark of Blackwell Science Ltd,
registered at the United Kingdom
Trade Marks Registry

DISTRIBUTORS

Marston Book Services Ltd
PO Box 269
Abingdon, Oxon OX14 4YN
(Orders: Tel: 01235 465500
       Fax: 01235 465555)

USA
Blackwell Science, Inc.
Commerce Place
350 Main Street
Malden, MA 02148 5018
(Orders: Tel: 800 759 6102
       781 388 8250
       Fax: 781 388 8255)

Canada
Login Brothers Book Company
324 Saulteaux Crescent
Winnipeg, Manitoba R3J 3T2
(Orders: Tel: 204 837 2987)

Australia
Blackwell Science Pty Ltd
54 University Street
Carlton, Victoria 3053
(Orders: Tel: 3 9347 0300
       Fax: 3 9347 5001)

Catalogue records for this title
are available from the British Library
and the Library of Congress

ISBN 0-632-05083-7

For further information on
Blackwell Science, visit our website:
www.blackwell-science.com

Contents

Preface

The aim of this book has been to share the experience and lessons I have learned from 10 years of treating headache patients in a specialist clinic. Much of this time has been working alongside doctors from primary care giving me an insight into the advantages and limitations of general practice. I make no apology for describing a detailed approach— only by knowing the rules can the rules be broken. I have outlined a tried and tested technique for diagnosis and management of migraine which can be adapted to suit the reader's own approach. Information in each chapter is cross-referenced to other relevant chapters, enabling readers to skip chapters that are irrelevant to their needs.

Primary care is undergoing a further round of changes with development of primary care groups which, by encompassing a broader spectrum of healthcare professionals, will enable greater delegation of duties. This approach is particularly suited to migraine, a condition that often involves opticians, dentists, physiotherapists, etc. I hope that this text will provide useful information for everyone involved in patient care.

Acknowledgements

This book would never have been written without guidance and encouragement from Dr Nat Blau and Dr Marcia Wilkinson, from the City of London Migraine Clinic, who set me on an unexpected path to a career in migraine. Thanks are also due to GPs Dr Bill Hall and Dr Jane Lindsay, to Dr Robert Willcox, an occupational health physician, to Dr Tim Steiner, The Princess Margaret Migraine Clinic, Charing Cross Hospital, London; Dr John Edmeads, Sunnybrook Health Science Centre, Toronto, Canada; and to the staff and members of Migraine Action Association. Finally, a big thank you to all my patients.

CHAPTER 1

Introduction

I think a lot of people don't go and see their GPs when they have migraines because it is trivialized in so many people's minds. It is surprising how many people think: 'it's a headache, it's only a headache.' But it isn't, it is much more than a headache.

Patient comment

Fewer than 2% of the population say that they have never had a headache. Fortunately, most headaches have an obvious cause such as a sinus infection or overindulgence in alcohol. Such headaches rarely last longer than a few hours and, if treatment is necessary, symptoms readily respond to a couple of painkillers bought from the chemist.

But migraine is more than just a headache. Additional symptoms of nausea, vomiting, photophobia and phonophobia can make it impossible for the sufferer to keep going during an attack—which, in some cases, may last 2 or 3 days. Despite the obvious resultant disability and the improved identification of migraine, direct costs related to diagnosis and treatment represent only a fraction of the direct costs related to less prevalent conditions such as asthma. This discrepancy can be attributed to the fact that, unlike asthma, migraine is not considered a life-threatening condition.

What has been missing from the equation is data on morbidity related to migraine. Recent research addressing this issue has highlighted the impact that migraine can have on the health of a significant number of sufferers. Migraine can affect relationships, restrict social life and wreak havoc on career plans. As Jo Liddell, past director of the Migraine Action Association (formerly the British Migraine Association) once said: 'Migraine may not be life-threatening but it is certainly quality-of-life threatening'.

In addition, migraine results in an indirect financial burden to society. Since the highest prevalence of migraine affects those in their peak years of productivity, absence from work related to migraine is associated with substantial indirect costs. For a population of 37.8 million adults of working age in the UK, using an estimated migraine prevalence of 10%, indirect costs due to lost productivity amount to nearly £1200 million each year [1].

1

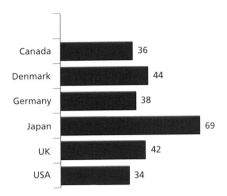

Fig. 1.1 Percentage of migraineurs who have never consulted a doctor for migraine.

Unfortunately, despite increasing awareness of the true prevalence of migraine and its associated disability, the condition remains underdiagnosed and undertreated in the community. Between 30 and 70% of migraine sufferers have never consulted a doctor for migraine (Fig. 1.1). The average group practice might see only 80 new consultations for migraine per year and 20 patients for repeated follow-up [2]. In terms of numbers consulting per GP, figures vary considerably. A sample of 650 GPs who recorded a diagnosis of migraine in any of their patients to the year ending May 1998, suggests that each GP saw an average of 27 migraine patients and prescribed medication for 19 of these [3]. Although the majority of people with migraine cope just with over-the-counter treatments, some experience periods of frequent, severe attacks. Why do so few sufferers seek medical advice? Reasons given include the belief that there are no effective treatments, or that migraine is a condition they should be able to cope with, as their parents did. Typically, they will only make an appointment to see a doctor when attacks become more frequent or when symptoms change.

But there is no need for silent suffering. In the last few decades, a better understanding of the science of migraine has led to the development of revolutionary treatments specific to the condition. Patients with migraine can now take advantage of better management strategies. Despite this, many of those who consult their doctor still fail to get the help that they need and many do not bother to return for follow-up. A survey of the Migraine Action Association revealed that 21% of members felt that their GP either did not understand the problem, or did not take them seriously. Neither are patients always given the correct diagnosis (Fig. 1.2).

Part of the problem is that many doctors do not enjoy treating mi-

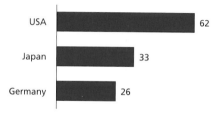

Fig. 1.2 Migraine: a missed diagnosis? The percentage of consulters with migraine receiving diagnosis of migraine.

graine, considering it a difficult problem, particularly since there is no cure. Attitude to headache consultations is not helped by popular mythology representing migraine patients as neurotic and demanding. My experience working with doctors from general practice is that dissatisfaction with treating headache patients often stems from lack of knowledge. This is not surprising when you consider that the average undergraduate teaching on headache amounts to less than 1 h over 5 years of training.

Consulting rates for migraine rose by over 40% in the 10 years between 1981 and 1992, a figure which is set to increase. Like it or not, doctors will have to treat more migraine patients. In writing this book, I aim to provide doctors and other healthcare workers with a basic knowledge of the diagnosis and management of migraine. Further experience can be gained from the patients—who were certainly the source of most of my own knowledge. Although I work in a specialist clinic, I believe strongly that migraine is a condition that can, and should, be managed in general practice. Primary care physicians develop a unique relationship with their patients, often over many years. This can provide the physician with a better understanding of provoking stresses and the impact of any resultant disability related to migraine for each individual. This personal knowledge of patients also helps the physician to cope with an important limitation of primary care—time.

Cost considerations are of particular concern in modern practice. Although migraine cannot be cured, it can be controlled with a combination of drug and non-drug treatments, which need not be expensive. Using a flexible approach, treatments should be reviewed and adapted at regular intervals.

Migraine is shrouded in myths and misconceptions. Lack of knowledge can make it a frustrating condition to treat. Armed with a better understanding of the disorder, even sceptics may begin to find that migraine can be satisfying to treat—particularly when patients return to thank you. There is also the added benefit of knowing that successful

1

therapy not only reduces the burden of migraine to the individual. It also reduces the burden to society.

References

1 Data on file. Zeneca Pharmaceuticals.
2 McCormick A, Fleming D, Charlton J. *Morbidity Statistics for General Practice: Fourth National Study 1991–1995*. London, HMSO, 1995.
3 MediPlus®. UK Primary Care Database.

CHAPTER 2

Migraine: from Past to Present

Migraine defined

The term 'migraine' was originally derived from the Greek word *hemicrania* meaning half (*hemi*) skull (*crania*). Translated into French, this became *migraine*.

It is tempting to believe that migraine is a modern affliction, triggered by the stresses and strains of 20th century life. Such a misconception is easily shattered, as migraine has been known to afflict mankind for centuries, from the first historic writings.

Zeus, the father of the Greek Gods, had such a severe headache that he required a surgical operation. As his skull was opened by Vulcan, so the Goddess of Wisdom was born.

Hippocrates, in around 400 BC, gave one of the earliest accounts of migraine. He described a shining light in the eye which was followed by severe pain in the temples, spreading to affect the entire head and neck. Hippocrates noted that the pain of migraine was often restricted to one side of the head and was associated with nausea and vomiting.

Aretaeus of Cappadocia, at the end of the first century AD, also wrote that the pain of migraine was usually restricted to one half of the head. He gives a particularly accurate and vivid description of an attack:

> In certain cases the parts on the right side, or those on the left solely (are affected), so far that a separate temple, or ear, or one eyebrow, or one eye, or the nose which divides the fact into two equal parts. The pain does not pass this limit, but remains in the half of the head. This is called heterocrania, an illness by no means mild, even though it intermits, and although it appears to be slight. For if at any time it sets in acutely, it occasions unseemly and dreadful symptoms: nausea, vomiting of bilious matters, collapse of the patient, or if more light and not deadly, it becomes chronic; there is much torpor, heaviness of the head, anxiety and weariness. For they flee the light; the darkness soothes their disease. Nor can they bear readily to look upon or hear anything disagreeable. Their sense of smell is vitiated. Neither does anything agreeable to smell delight

them and they also have an aversion to foetid things. The patients moreover are weary of life and wish to die.

2

The causes of migraine

In ancient times, headache sufferers were believed to be possessed by demons—a belief which remained popular for many centuries.

Hippocrates recognized that the psyche played an important part, with anger and sadness triggering headache that could only be relieved by calming the soul. In his vast treatise on medicine, the Corpus Hippocraticum, Hippocrates considered that disease was due to an imbalance in the bodily humours with headache due to toxic blood released by the gall bladder. He shows remarkable insight into the cause of the pain, writing that it was induced in the blood vessels surrounding the skull and meninges.

By the 17th century, it was realized that migraine could be brought on by drinking wine, overeating, lying in the sun, passion, sexual activity and too much sleep. Sufferers were advised to lead the joyless existence of a life without wine, sun or sex and had to avoid any emotion. They were treated by the application of leeches and the letting of blood to rid the body of noxious elements.

Thomas Willis (1621–1675) was the first to draw attention to the vascular theory of migraine. In his book published in 1672, he included a treatise entitled *De Cephalalgia*. In this, Willis shows an extraordinary awareness of many of the triggering factors of migraine: 'changes of the season, atmospheric states, the great aspects of the sun and moon, violent passions, and errors in diet.' He also suggested that migraine was caused by vasodilatation in the meninges, further stating that symptoms were related to slowly ascending spasms beginning in the peripheral ends of the nerves.

Much was written about migraine during the 18th century with demons continuing to remain a popular cause of headache. However, it was noticed that more women suffered from migraine than men. The term 'uterine megrim' was coined by Robert Whytt who believed that headaches arose from the womb, a theory which remained popular until the middle of the last century. Others thought that a 'nervous temperament' was the cause, or blamed constipation.

Edward Liveing published the treatise *On Megrim, Sick-Headache and Some Allied Disorders* in 1873, challenging the vascular theory (Fig. 2.1). He recognized the many clinical presentations of migraine and developed the theory of 'nerve-storms'. He related migraine to epilepsy, both of which were thought to be caused by discharges in the central

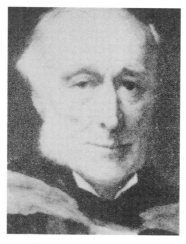

Fig. 2.1 Edward Liveing: the first person to consider a nonvascular origin. Courtesy of Dr J. Edmeads.

nervous system. William Gowers was a further advocate of this neural theory, and expanded on Liveing's thesis in the late 19th century.

In 1938, John Graham and Harold Wolff published a paper on the 'Mechanism of migraine headache and the action of ergotamine tartrate'. They demonstrated that ergotamine acts in migraine by constricting blood vessels and used this finding to support the vascular theory of migraine.

Since that time both the vascular and neuronal theories have remained hotly debated and have now been combined into the neurovascular theory of migraine. Migraine research has progressed rapidly over the last decade but, although our understanding of the condition has increased, no single theory has managed to account for all the features of migraine. It is recognized that in a migraine attack genetic, constitutional and environmental factors combine with hormonal and biochemical changes to produce measurable effects throughout the body which are not seen in other types of headache. However, the mechanism of these changes remains a mystery—at least for the present.

Remedies for headache

One of the oldest headache remedies, dating from about 8000 BC is recounted in this Sumarian poem, the *Incantation of Eridu*:

> *Take the hair of a virgin kid*
> *Let a wise woman spin it on the right angle*

7

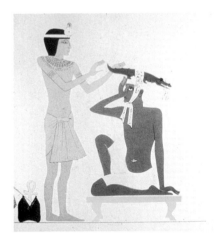

Fig. 2.2 Clay crocodile: an early cure for headache. Courtesy of Dr J. Edmeads.

And double it on the left
Bind twice with seven knots
Then perform the incantation of Eridu;
Bind therewith the head of the sick man
Bind therewith the neck of the sick man
Bind therewith his life
Cast the water of the incantation over him
That the headache may ascend to heaven

The Egyptian Ebers Papyrus, dating from around 1200 BC also contains an ancient remedy for migraine: 'bind a clay crocodile, with a decorated eye and straw in its mouth, to the head of the patient using a strip of fine linen upon which has been inscribed the names of the gods, and he shall pray' (Fig. 2.2).

Both these treatments may have been effective as external pressure on distended temporal arteries has been shown to alleviate the pain.

A less pleasant ancient treatment was trepanation, the removal of a segment of bone, seen in Neolithic skulls dating from 7000 BC. Despite the invasiveness of this procedure, patients appear to have survived as many of the trepanned skulls show evidence of healing. It is thought that this was performed in order to release the demons and evil spirits trapped inside the head, which were responsible for the headache. Given the questionable merits of such treatment, it is astounding that trepanation was still being recommended as a migraine treatment by some 17th century physicians, notably William Harvey.

Some ancient therapies are still used today. The benefits of acupuncture were recorded in *The Yellow Emperor's Text of Internal Medi-*

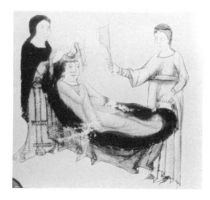

Fig. 2.3 The medieval treatment of headache. Courtesy of Dr J. Edmeads.

cine, which dates from between the eighth and third centuries BC. Hippocrates recommended an extract of willow bark for pain relief. Modern medicine has shown us that the active ingredient of willow bark is salicylic acid—popularly known today, in its refined form, as aspirin.

Galen of Pergamum, in the second century AD, considered that migraine was caused by an excess of body fluid entering through the gastrointestinal system and irritating the brain. Bloodletting and purging were the recommended management.

Other Greek physicians experimented with more pharmacological remedies. Discoride (77 AD) found the extract of the ruta plant to be effective. The active ingredient, rutin, is known to lower blood pressure.

During medieval times diverse concoctions were recommended, such as an English headache tonic containing elderberry juice, cow's brain, vinegar and goat dung. Opium and vinegar solutions became popular throughout Europe, applied to the head using a drug-soaked poultice (Fig. 2.3). It is thought that the vinegar opened the pores of the skin enabling the opium to be rapidly absorbed. Perhaps this is the origin of Jack's treatment in the nursery rhyme:

Jack and Jill went up the hill to fetch a pail of water
Jack fell down and broke his crown and Jill came tumbling after
Then up Jack got and home did trot as fast as he could caper
He went to bed to mend his head with vinegar and brown paper

In South America, the Incas dripped coca juice into a scalp incision and the American Indians used a combination of extracts of willow bark and beaver testes. Both these treatments are likely to have been effective as they contain natural analgesics—cocaine and salicylic acid.

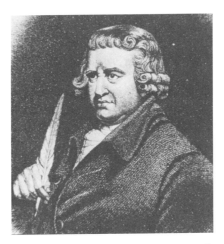

Fig. 2.4 Erasmus Darwin: proposed headache relief by centrifugation. Courtesy of Dr J. Edmeads.

Samuel Andre Tissot, a Swiss neurologist, published a textbook of neurology at the end of the 17th century which included detailed descriptions of several different types of headache. He referred to coffee as an effective migraine treatment but also stated that if coffee was drunk on a regular basis, headache would be triggered when the coffee was withdrawn.

By the 18th century, treatment had progressed further. Erasmus Darwin, grandfather of Charles Darwin, suggested that centrifugal force could be used to force blood out of the brain (Fig. 2.4). Such a centrifuge was developed by Harold Wolff over 150 years later. It did not prove popular with patients!

Gradually more sensible approaches to migraine therapy were identified. In 1881, the German doctor Eulenberg recommended ergot alkaloids. In 1888 William Gowers revisited the practice of the identification and avoidance of lifestyle triggers. He wrote: 'If any error in mode of life or defect in general health can be traced, the removal of this is the most and most essential step in treatment'. Gowers also defined therapeutic goals and was the first to consider prophylactic treatment with drugs to render attacks less frequent (Fig. 2.5). For acute treatment, he developed 'Gower's Mixture' containing bromide and cannabis. William Osler recommended cannabis but also noted that the treatments containing chemicals with similar properties to paracetamol and aspirin were effective.

In 1897, Dr Felix Hoffman invented aspirin—a drug which has stood the test of time and remains a standard treatment for migraine to this day.

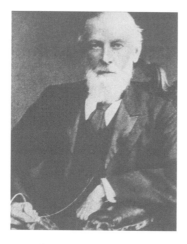

Fig. 2.5 William Gowers: an advocate of the neurogenic theory. Courtesy of Dr J. Edmeads.

By 1925, the Swiss chemist Rothlin isolated the vasoconstrictor ergotamine, which rapidly became a popular treatment for migraine. There was little further progress until the mid-1970s when it was noted that gastric stasis inhibited the absorption of oral analgesics during migraine attacks. It was found that this effect could be reversed by using metoclopramide, a pro-kinetic antiemetic. This combination of analgesics and metoclopramide, or a similar drug domperidone, is still recommended when simple analgesics alone are ineffective.

The last 20 years

Although there have been few advances in prophylactic treatment, the late 20th century has heralded a revolution in acute migraine management. Elucidation of the role of the neurotransmitter serotonin in the migraine process, and the identification of specific serotonin, or 5-hydroxytryptamine (5HT), receptors have led to the development of the most modern acute therapies, the 5HT1 agonists. Although they have their limitations, they represent a major advance in the pharmacotherapy of migraine. Undoubtedly, given the present flurry of research, even more exciting advances await us in the 21st century.

Developments in services

Until recently, provision of care has been limited. The current surge of interest associated with the development of specific migraine drugs has highlighted a more accurate prevalence of migraine, the associated dis-

2

ability and the need for better care. The majority of patients with migraine can be managed exclusively in general practice. Referrals, when necessary, are mostly to neurologists, who may or may not have a specific interest in the condition.

An advance in management has been the development of specialist migraine clinics. During the 1950s Macdonald Critchley set up part-time headache clinics at King's College Hospital and at the National Hospital for Nervous Diseases. Marcia Wilkinson followed with a clinic at the women's hospital, the Elizabeth Garrett Anderson. Dr Michael Hay, a GP, opened a clinic in Birmingham. Dr Vera Walker opened a clinic in Bournemouth, with the help of Dr Peter Wilson. Dr Judith Hockaday raised awareness of the problem of headaches in children with a paediatric clinic in Oxford.

More recently, the Migraine Trust has helped to set up other clinics around the UK. Most of these are linked to neurological services and are funded by the NHS. The City of London Migraine Clinic was originally funded by the Migraine Trust when it opened in 1970 (first known as the City Migraine Clinic) but became an independent medical charity in 1980. It is the only clinic in the UK to provide a nation-wide free service for referring primary care physicians. The founding of the City of London Migraine Clinic heralded a new approach to migraine. It was the first dedicated clinic to remain open throughout the working week and was the first to treat patients during acute migraine attacks. The clinic was set up in the City to serve the influx of City workers, many of whom were likely to develop migraine. This provided a research population for studying mechanisms of migraine and for testing new treatments. The success of the clinic is apparent from the fact that it has been used as a model for similar services around the world.

Another advantage of specialist services is that staff have more time and specific expertise. They can provide a more individual approach to management based on a broader understanding of the treatments available. As research centres, invaluable information can be gained into the mechanism and management of migraine and other headaches.

Developments in the structure of research

Headache research became formalized with the inception of the International Headache Society, founded in London on 23 September 1982. Plans for the development of the Society had been underway for several years. One successful aim has been to provide an international forum for everyone interested in headache with an exchange of research results, presented at international meetings held every second year. The

Society produces its own journal, *Cephalalgia*. Ten issues are published each year. Teaching is high on the list of Society aims, with the emphasis on educating doctors from all over the world but particularly those from countries with minimal facilities for headache management. The Society has expanded over the years, acting as an 'umbrella' organization for national societies and incorporating national lay groups. Publications aimed at improving research included a classification and diagnostic criteria for over 150 different headaches and guidelines for controlled clinical trials in migraine [1], tension-type headache [2] and cluster headache [3]. The need for improvements in headache management led to the recent publication *Organization and Delivery of Services to Headache Patients* [4]. This document aims to provide a model for use by local headache societies and doctors in their attempts to influence authorities to provide better standards of care.

Changes in primary care

Although headache is a common complaint in primary care, lack of education and time mean that many GPs report difficulties in diagnosis and management. This was highlighted by the results of a survey of 600 international primary care physicians who were questioned in the ADITUS Primary Care Research Study [5]. Of this group, 75–80% reported that they found migraine a difficult condition to treat. It is not surprising that the most satisfactory consultations, both for the doctors and their patients, are those in which the doctors feel that they have a sound understanding of the problem and can provide a solution.

Better education

Education is an important key to this and it is unfortunate that migraine is very low on the list of priorities in undergraduate training. In recent years, more literature has become available and more postgraduate courses are run. It is important to note that patients want more than just drug therapy. More than 70% of patients attending The City of London Migraine Clinic, a specialist centre, are already using 'triptans', often effectively. These patients often request more information about the migraine process, how drugs work, and how they can prevent and treat attacks without resorting to drugs.

Research in general practice

Another positive aspect has been the involvement of primary care physicians in trials of drug therapies for migraine and clinical epidemiology. More research into the identification of migraine in primary care, and other aspects of management, is also underway.

Audit

Audit has an increasingly important role medical practice. Audit of migraine can identify the extent of the problem in general practice, misdiagnosis and treatment issues as well as merits and deficiencies in care. These results can be used to develop better local services.

Improving care in general practice

Specialist services are limited by cost and a shortfall in consultant neurologists. Further, with the development of primary care groups, the emphasis of management is now focused on general practice. In the case of migraine, recent advances have highlighted the problem of migraine, leading to improved undergraduate and postgraduate education. This should result in better competence and confidence in diagnosis and management, avoiding the unnecessary referral for the patient who is worried about a brain tumour. Time limitations can be overcome by involving nursing staff and other healthcare workers linked to general practice. Patients can also be directed to self-help organizations for further information about their headache (see Appendix A). Fewer referrals has a further consequence of conserving limited practice finances.

District guidelines, such as those used for epilepsy, could be developed for migraine and may well become necessary within the new NHS.

References

1 International Headache Society Committee on Clinical Trials in Migraine. Guidelines for controlled trials of drugs in migraine. First Edition. *Cephalalgia* 1991; 11: 3–12.
2 International Headache Society Committee on Clinical Trials. Guidelines for trials of drug treatments in tension-type headache. *Cephalalgia* 1995; 15: 165–79.
3 International Headache Society Committee on Clinical Trials in Cluster Headache. Guidelines for controlled trials of drugs in cluster headache. *Cephalalgia* 1995; 15: 452–62.
4 Task force of the International Headache Society. Organization and delivery of services to headache patients. *Cephalalgia* 1997; 17: 702–10.
5 ADITUS Primary Care Research Study conducted by Taylor Nelson AGB plc. Data on file, Zeneca Pharmaceuticals, 1996.

CHAPTER 3

Who Gets Migraine?

Studies suggest that migraine affects at least 10–15% of the population. Considering a working population of about 38 million adults, this amounts to about 3.8–5.7 million people in the UK. However, this is only an estimate as it is difficult to assess the exact incidence and prevalence of the condition. Part of the reason for this is that so few people with migraine visit the doctor, and therefore population-based market-research studies have been necessary.

Another problem is that accepted diagnostic criteria for clinical trials in migraine were only introduced in 1988. Studies undertaken before this date used inconsistent criteria making it impossible to compare results. Several studies have been undertaken using the new criteria have shown consistently similar results.

Incidence

There have been no prospective studies assessing incidence. This is unfortunate as recall bias is a considerable problem in migraine. One recent study of children identified with migraine and followed to middle age showed that many of them had forgotten that they had experienced attacks with aura as children [1]. Therefore data from retrospective studies should be viewed with caution, although they do give an indication of the problem.

A study of patients attending the City of London Migraine Clinic showed that, in both sexes, migraine began in childhood and adolescence with an earlier peak incidence for boys than for girls. Incidence then declines over time in both sexes. At least 90% of the population with migraine have their first attack before the age of 40.

Larger population-based retrospective studies have produced similar results [2] but only prospective studies will confirm these findings.

Prevalence studies (Fig. 3.1)

Migraine prevalence varies with sex, age, socio-economic status and race. Prevalence is difficult to measure as migraine is an episodic condition with attacks varying in frequency from year to year. Most stud-

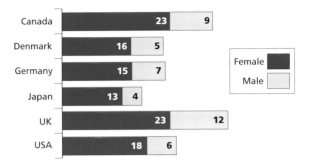

Fig. 3.1 One-year prevalence of migraine (%).

ies have assessed 1-year prevalence, i.e. the number of people experiencing at least one known attack migraine in the previous year.

Prevalence rates from European and American studies are remarkably similar. In Denmark, 1000 men and women aged between 25 and 64 were interviewed about their general health and headaches [3]. The researchers found that 8% of men and 25% of women questioned had had an attack of migraine at some time in their lives. One-year prevalence was reported as 5% for men and 16% for women.

A survey in America set out to analyse the results of a questionnaire sent to 15 000 households. Replies were received from 63% of people aged between 12 and 80. From this group, 6% of men and 18% of women reported having one or more migraine headaches each year [2].

In the UK, a study of workers in an ICI chemicals factory identified ≈23% of female employees who had experienced a migraine attack in the preceding year, compared with 12% of male employees [4].

Migraine is reported to be on the increase. One American study reported a 60% increase in migraine during the 1980s. In Finland, a study of 7-year-olds with migraine showed a threefold increase in prevalence over two decades [5]. It is not known whether these figures reflect a true increase in prevalence or are the result of better recognition and reporting of migraine. It is worth noting that the Finnish study was undertaken by the same researcher in the same city and in the same school 22 years after the initial study.

Sex

During the reproductive years, migraine affects more women than men in a ratio of about 3 : 1. Hormonal changes in women are the obvious reason for this difference between the sexes, which could also account for the fact that until puberty, migraine is equally prevalent in boys

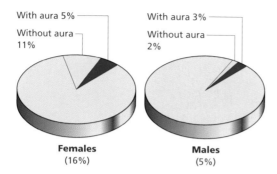

With aura 5%

Without aura
11%

With aura 3%

Without aura
2%

Females
(16%)

Males
(5%)

3

Fig. 3.2 Type of migraine. Based on data from Rasmussen BK. Epidemiology of headache. *Cephalalgia* 1995; 15: 45–68.

and girls. However, hormones cannot be the sole factor as the gender differences persist past the menopause.

Type of migraine (Fig. 3.2)

Women are more likely to have migraine without aura than migraine with aura, with 1-year prevalence rates of 11% and 5%, respectively. Lifetime prevalence suggests a male to female ratio of 1 : 7 for migraine without aura. For men, there is little difference between the type of migraine with a 1-year prevalence of migraine without aura and migraine with aura of 2% and 3%, respectively. This difference in the type of migraine may reflect hormonal differences as migraine triggered by oestrogen withdrawal in women is typically without aura.

Age (Fig. 3.3)

Even though migraine starts in the young, it may not become a problem until later life. The peak prevalence for migraine without aura is early to mid-forties for women and men.

Migraine usually improves in later life in both sexes, although a few continue to have attacks. The reason for this decline in prevalence is unknown, although it has been postulated that it could relate to a reduced vascular response with advancing years.

Race

Studies from African and Asian countries have reportedly shown a much lower prevalence of migraine. However, these differences may reflect varying methodology and social attitude to headache. Alternatively, a

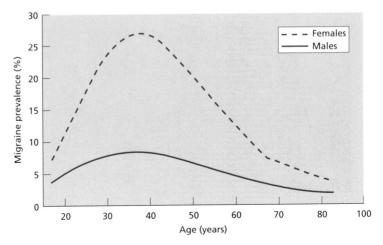

Fig. 3.3 Age- and sex-specific prevalence of migraine. Reprinted with permission from Advanstar Communications Inc. as reprinted from *Neurology* 1993; 43 (Suppl. 3): 6. *Neurology*® is a registered trademark of the American Academy of Neurology.

difference in genetic susceptibility to migraine could be the underlying factor.

Socio-economic status

It has often been thought that migraine sufferers were more intelligent than non-sufferers and of higher social class. This myth was dispelled when it was found that people who have had more years of education are more likely to seek treatment from a doctor. In fact migraine affects people from all walks of life regardless of race, intelligence or social class. There is even some epidemiological evidence to suggest that migraine is more prevalent in the lower social classes. Reasons for this could include a difference in occupation between the social classes (e.g. greater exposure to toxic fumes in manual jobs), increased stress, poor living conditions and inadequate healthcare resources. Despite this higher prevalence, people with low income seem less likely to seek medical advice.

Prognosis (Fig. 3.4)

The only longitudinal study of migraine over 40 years, based on a cohort of 73 children with migraine, confirms the variability of migraine over time [1]. A total of 51% still reported migraine at the 40-year fol-

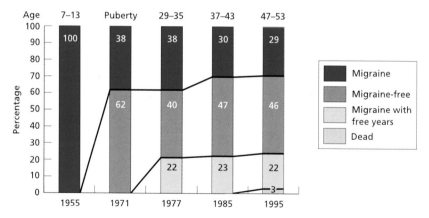

Fig. 3.4 The prognosis for school children with pronounced migraine during a 40-year follow-up period. Reproduced with permission from Bille BA. A 40-year follow-up of school children with migraine. *Cephalalgia* 1996; 17: 488–91.

low-up: 29% had continued to suffer from migraine, at least annually, without remission and 22% still had migraine but had experienced one or more migraine-free periods of at least 2 years, the average being 10 years. Three per cent had died and 46% were free of migraine—23% having been permanently free since puberty. The prognosis was better for boys than for girls. In general, attacks in adulthood were reported as being less frequent but of similar intensity to childhood migraine.

Migraine genes?

Why should any particular person develop migraine? There is undoubtedly a familial link but whether migraine is a learned response or a true genetic condition is the subject of debate.

Twin studies have been the obvious means of identifying the true cause but most have been subject to recall bias and selection bias that make interpretation of the results difficult. The coexistence of several different types of migraine in the same person makes it difficult to study the genetics of specific types of migraine. Further, studies tend to be undertaken on subjects with relatively frequent attacks. What about the individual who has only ever had one or two migraines? Even with these limitations, no twin study has shown 100% concordance. This means that, although a genetic component may be present, environmental factors are important.

Some types of migraine may have a greater genetic basis than others. The extremely rare condition of familial hemiplegic migraine has been the focus of intense research culminating in the discovery of a gene assigned to chromosome 19 found in about 50% of affected families tested [6]. Since some authorities believe that familial hemiplegic migraine is part of the migraine spectrum, ongoing research has aimed to identify the involvement of this gene in the more usual forms of migraine. The same locus has been implicated for migraine with and without aura, as have genes on chromosomes 1, 4 and 13. Other chromosomes are probably also involved.

What is the inherited factor? It is most likely to be the threshold to attacks. This model means that it is possible for every individual to experience migraine provided they have sufficient triggers to cross the attack threshold. Those who inherit a lower threshold require fewer triggers to initiate an attack. This would also account for the increased prevalence of migraine in women, by virtue of their additional hormonal trigger during the reproductive years. It would also fit with the research that suggests that the genetic loci are responsible for cerebral calcium channels. Impairment of normal function of these calcium channels may facilitate the initiation of attacks, i.e. be responsible for the attack threshold. What it does not explain is why some people should develop migraine with aura, some without aura and others with both; or how the type of migraine can change with time in the same person.

It is worth considering that other factors may determine the familial pattern of migraine, in particular learned response. Children learn patterns of behaviour from their parents—especially from their mother—which is likely to include learning a means of coping with headache. As doctors, we often provide reinforcement of this behaviour with our drugs, when motivation for change may be a more successful long-term option.

References

1　Bille BA. 40-year follow-up of school children with migraine. *Cephalalgia* 1997; 17: 488–91.
2　Stewart WF, Linet MS, Celentano DD *et al.* Age- and sex-specific incidence rates of migraine with and without visual aura. *Am J Epidemiol* 1991; 134: 1111–20.
3　Rasmussen BK. Epidemiology of headache. *Cephalalgia* 1995; 15: 45–68.
4　Mountstephen AH, Harrison RK. A study of migraine and its effects in a working population. *Occup Med* 1995; 45: 311–7.
5　Sillanpää M, Anttila P. Increasing prevalence of headache in 7-year-old schoolchildren. *Headache* 1996; 36: 466–70.
6　May A, Ophoff RA, Terwindt GM *et al.* Familial hemiplegic migraine locus on 19p13 is involved in the common forms of migraine with and without aura. *Hum Genet* 1995; 96: 604–8.

CHAPTER 4

What is Migraine?

It might not be a life-threatening disease but it is debilitating. It affects our lives and the lives of our families. It starts to control us. I've fought back saying 'No, I'm going to control it' and that's the only way I've been able to survive ...

Patient comment

4

Symptoms (Fig. 4.1)

The name 'migraine' is derived from the Greek word *hemicrania* meaning a one-sided headache. But migraine is more than just a headache and the headache is not necessarily the major symptom. During the attack concentration is limited and each task takes twice as long—if it is possible to tackle it at all. Sufferers often have to rest in a quiet,

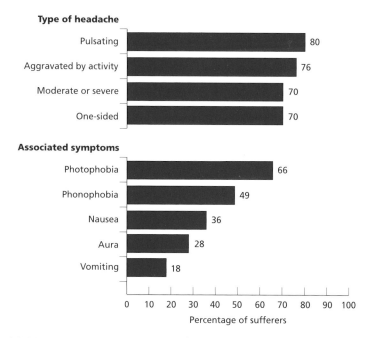

Fig. 4.1 Migraine symptoms. From Micieli G. Suffering in silence. In: *Migraine: A Brighter Future*. Edmeads J, ed. Worthing, Cambridge Medical Publications, 1993: 1–7.

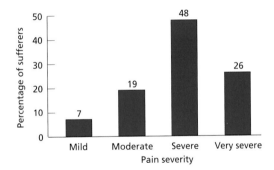

Fig. 4.2 Severity of headache pain during attacks. From Henry P, Michel P, Bouchat B *et al.* A nationwide survey of migraine in France: prevalence and clinical features in adults. *Cephalalgia* 1992; 12: 229–37.

darkened room until the symptoms ease. Many are anorexic and nauseous but, despite this, may need to eat. Gastric stasis is a feature with particular clinical relevance as absorption of oral medication may be reduced, especially if treatment is delayed. Sometimes an attack ends with vomiting but in most cases the headache improves after a good sleep.

Severity (Fig. 4.2)

Despite the low consultation rate for migraine, population studies suggest that around two-thirds of migraineurs questioned report severe or very severe attacks.

Frequency (Fig. 4.3)

Population studies show that the average frequency is eight to 12 attacks per year. In reality, the frequency of migraine varies considerably

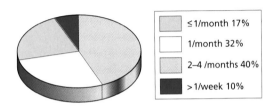

Fig. 4.3 Frequency of attacks. From Henry P, Michel P, Bouchat B *et al.* A nationwide survey of migraine in France: prevalence and clinical features in adults. *Cephalalgia* 1992; 12: 229–37.

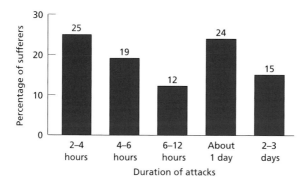

Fig. 4.4 Duration of attacks. From Henry P, Michel P, Bouchat B *et al*. A nationwide survey of migraine in France: prevalence and clinical features in adults. *Cephalalgia* 1992; 12: 229–37.

both between individuals and in the same person. Attacks may come once or twice a month during a bad patch but a few unlucky people might have a spell of attacks occurring once or twice a week. This could be followed by a gap of several months or even years without an attack, for no apparent reason. In general, attacks become less frequent after the age of 55, although this is not always the case. If patients report attacks regularly occurring more often than once a week, it is likely that they have an additional headache or are at risk of medication misuse headache.

Timing of attacks

Migraine typically starts in the morning with attacks present on waking or commencing soon after. This has important therapeutic implications as oral treatment is more likely to be ineffective if an attack is fully developed on waking, particularly if associated with severe nausea or vomiting.

Duration (Fig. 4.4)

The headache of a migraine usually eases within 24 h of starting but can last anything from part of a day to 3 days. Often it takes another day or so to get back to normal as symptoms of tiredness and feeling 'washed out' remain even after the headache has gone. A few people feel extra well after an attack—possibly due to relief that the attack is over.

Children typically have shorter attacks lasting only a few hours or even less.

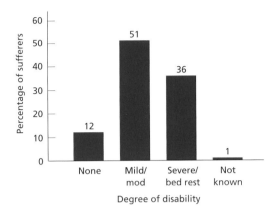

Fig. 4.5 Migraine disability. From Stewart WF, Lipton RB, Celentano DD *et al.* Prevalence of migraine headache in the United States. *JAMA* 1992; 267: 64–69. Stewart WF, Shechter A, Lipton RB. Migraine heterogeneity. *Neurology* 1994; 44 (Suppl. 4): 24–39.

Disability (Fig. 4.5)

Migraine can be associated with considerable disability. Several studies carried out in different countries show that migraine impaired normal function in more than three-quarters of sufferers. About one-third have to lie down during a migraine with obvious impact on work and other daily activities.

Defining migraine

As you can see, the term 'migraine' covers a broad spectrum of symptoms that can be different in different individuals and even vary in the same individual for separate attacks. For some it is just a 'sick' headache while for others, the headache is preceded by visual aura. But more specific definitions are necessary to make a diagnosis.

Migraine has been defined as 'an episodic headache lasting part of a day up to three days associated with visual and/or gastrointestinal disturbance and general malaise'. This provides a useful overview of the main symptoms that make up a migraine attack. Episodicity is an important feature as there is complete freedom from symptoms between attacks; daily headaches are not migraine.

With a view to standardizing definitions for all headaches, including migraine, a committee was formed from members of the International Headache Society (IHS) in the mid-1980s. This led to the development of an extensive classification of the different headaches which was published in 1988 and which runs to 97 pages [1]. This classification is generally followed throughout this text.

Fortunately, an in-depth knowledge of every variety of headache is unnecessary as some varieties are much more common than others. In clinical practice patients present with symptoms of two main subtypes of migraine which differ only in their presence or absence of an 'aura'. About 70% of migraineurs experience attacks of **migraine without aura** (formerly known as common migraine) and 10% have **migraine with aura** (formerly known as classical migraine). About 20% have both types of attacks. Fewer than 1% of attacks are of aura alone with no headache ensuing.

Migraine without aura

The IHS definition of migraine without aura is:
> an idiopathic, recurring headache disorder manifesting in attacks lasting 4–72 hours. Typical characteristics of headache are unilateral location, pulsating quality, moderate or severe intensity, aggravation by routine physical activity, and association with nausea, photo- and phonophobia.

Migraine with aura

The IHS definition of migraine with aura is:
> an idiopathic, recurring disorder manifesting with attacks of neurological symptoms unequivocally localizable to cerebral cortex or brain stem, usually gradually developed over 15–20 minutes and usually lasting less than 60 minutes. Headache, nausea and/or photophobia usually follow the neurological aura symptoms directly or after a free interval of less than an hour. The headache usually lasts 4–72 hours.

Patients who experience the visual disturbances of the aura are often afraid of permanently losing their vision. Strokes and brain tumours are also common fears. Fortunately such sinister causes and sequelae are rare. In the case of strokes and tumours, other symptoms are usually apparent and the headache is progressive. These, and other causes of headache, are discussed in more detail in later chapters.

The clinical picture of migraine

Criteria are invaluable in order to standardize research but in clinical practice it is more helpful to make a diagnosis based on a picture of a

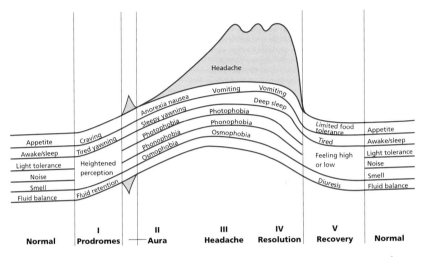

Fig. 4.6 Symptoms and signs during phases of complete classic migraine attacks. Reproduced with permission from Blau JN. Migraine: theories of pathogenesis. *Lancet* 1992; 339: 1202–7.

typical attack. An attack of migraine can be divided into several distinct phases, not all of which occur in every attack (Fig. 4.6).

Prodromes (Table 4.1)

Up to two-thirds of migraineurs experience warning symptoms of subtle changes in mood or behaviour which can precede attacks of both migraine with and without aura [2]. They are distinct from, and unrelated to, the aura. On average, they begin about 3 h before attacks of both migraine with and without aura but can occur anything up to 24–48 h earlier. They may not be noted by the patient unless attention is drawn to them by the doctor. Not infrequently, they are more apparent to the patient's family or partner or noted only retrospectively by the

Table 4.1 Typical prodromal symptoms (these should not be confused with aura and may precede attacks *with or without* aura).

Insidious onset
Last for several hours
Extreme lethargy and yawning
Depression or elation
Hunger and food cravings
Constipation or diarrhoea
Urinary frequency or retention
Dysphasia

patient. Symptoms slowly develop and are suggestive of hypothalamic disturbance. They include:

- *altered mental state*—irritability, feeling 'high' or 'low'—some patients describe feeling 'dangerously' well;
- *altered behaviour*—hyperactivity, obsessive behaviour, clumsiness, lethargy;
- *altered appearance*—pale, sunken eyes;
- *neurological symptoms*—tiredness or yawning, dysphasia, photo- and phonophobia, difficulty in focusing;
- *muscular aches and pains*;
- *alimentary symptoms*—craving for foods, anorexia, constipation, a craving for sweet foods may result in a desire to eat chocolate or other sweets, which are then incorrectly blamed as a cause of the attack;
- *symptoms related to fluid balance*—increased urinary frequency, thirst or fluid retention;
- *hypersensitivity*—to light, sound and smell.

In her book *Hotel du Lac*, Anita Brookner vividly describes prodromal symptoms which Edith experiences, the night before waking with a migraine:

> When, some 2 hours later, she sat down to dinner, she was aware that the lights were brighter, the room more alive with personalities, the tables full ... Edith was grateful for the warmth, the food, the service; she felt very tired, and thought that she would sleep soundly that night .... But sleep did not come easily .... When she awoke, rather later than usual, it was with the ancient and deadly foreknowledge that the day would be a write-off. Her broken night had left her with an aching head and an instinctive shrinking from both food and company. Minute noises seemed magnified: a trolley was wheeled vigorously along the corridor, and the high voices of the maids sounded unbearably piercing.

Prodromal symptoms do not necessarily develop into a full attack. Patients often state that they felt 'migrainous' but nothing more—perhaps they unconsciously avoid further migraine triggers and abort the attack.

Aura (Table 4.2; Fig. 4.7)

Symptoms of aura are localizable to the cerebral cortex or brain stem and gradually develop over several minutes, last under 1 hour, and usually resolve before the onset of headache. The typical duration of aura is 20 min. There may be a gap between the end of the aura and the start

Table 4.2 Typical aura symptoms.

Slow evolution over several minutes
Duration usually 10–30 min resolving within 1 h
Resolution typically before onset of headache
Visual symptoms (99% of auras)
    Positive (bright) scotoma
    Homonymous hemianapia (i.e. affecting the same hemifield of both
        eyes)
    Teichopsia/fortification spectra (i.e. gradually enlarging C shape with
        scintillating edges)
Sensory disturbance (31% of auras)
    Usually associated with visual symptoms
    Usually affects one arm spreading from fingers of hand up to face
    Leg is rarely affected
Speech (dysphasia, dysarthria, paraphasia) and motor disturbance (18%
        and 6% of auras, respectively)
    Usually associated with visual and/or sensory disturbance

of the headache. *Visual symptoms* are most common, experienced in 99% of auras and present in virtually every attack [3]. Typical visual aura is hemianopic but starts as a flickering, bright, zigzag line (tei-

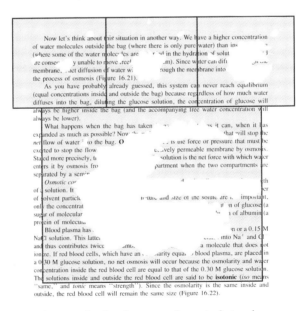

Fig. 4.7 Diagram showing the development of a typical visual aura commencing with a progressive central scotoma with crenellated edge. The scotoma gradually increases to fill most of the central field.

chopsia or fortification spectra) in the middle of the visual field, affecting central vision. This gradually progresses towards the periphery of one hemifield, often leaving a bright scotoma. As the semicircle enlarges and eventually disappears, the angle of the zigzag edges becomes wider and more irregular, and the rate of scintillation slows. Sometimes the progression halts partway across the visual field. *Sensory disturbance* is less common (31%) [3]. The typical sensory aura is unilateral, starting with pins and needles in one hand spreading up the arm to affect one side of the face and tongue. It is unusual for these symptoms to affect the legs. *Speech disturbance and motor symptoms* can also be present (18% and 6%, respectively) [3] but only in association with visual and/or sensory symptoms.

The gap

A gap between resolution of aura and onset of headache is common [4]. This interval is typically less than an hour, but can be longer. Alterations of mood, speech disturbance or a sensation of detachment from the environment have all been reported, symptoms which resemble prodromal symptoms.

Headache

The headache builds up gradually and lasts between 4 and 72 h. Attacks can be shorter, particularly if treated effectively. The headache is typically throbbing and one-sided, although it may swap sides during an attack, and can be bilateral. It can occur ipsilateral or contralateral to the side of the aura, if present. Severity can vary considerably.

Associated symptoms

Several of the following symptoms typically accompany headache:
* anorexia;
* nausea;
* vomiting;
* photophobia;
* phonophobia;
* osmophobia;
* general malaise.

Most sufferers sit or lie down with the curtains drawn, keeping still, since movement aggravates the pain and nausea. Despite anorexia, some patients find that eating carbohydrate helps.

Resolution

Other than with effective medication, the natural course of migraine is to resolve with sleep or vomiting [5].

Recovery

4

After the headache has gone, most migraineurs feel drained and 'hungover' for a further day [6]. Rarely, they feel very energetic and even euphoric. There is also a variable refractory phase directly following attacks during which further attacks cannot be triggered. In between attacks, they feel completely well, free from migraine symptoms.

Case study: migraine with aura

'I first notice visual symptoms, starting with blind spots varying from perhaps part of a letter missing on a page, looking like a misprint, to somebody's chin missing, or the loss of half my field of vision. This culminates in pulsating zigzag lines around objects giving the impression of the scene being viewed through a shattered mirror. My speech is affected—I can't put a sentence together. I feel confused and disorientated. This is the most distressing part of the migraine attack and it lasts about 15–20 minutes. Then my vision restores itself at the same time as a sick, one-sided pain starts in my head. This lasts for the rest of the day. I feel nauseous most of the time. When I was a child, I used to vomit. I usually feel very cold at the beginning of an attack and then later on, I get hot. If I am able to sleep, the headache has normally worn off by the time I wake up. I feel like I've been through a mangle for most of the next morning, and then I'm okay.'

The natural history of migraine

Migraine attacks can change over the course of time. The attacks often become more prolonged but less severe, unlike the short acute attacks usually seen in childhood. Migraine can convert from predominantly attacks of migraine with aura to migraine without aura and vice versa. Hormonal changes, such as those in pregnancy, can trigger attacks with marked focal symptoms. Similarly, the use of combined ethinyloestradiol/progestogen oral contraceptives can convert attacks previously without aura to those with aura. Removal of the hormonal trigger postpartum or by stopping the oral contraceptive pill does not necessarily cause attacks to revert to their former pattern.

But what do you say to the mother who asks about the prognosis for her child with migraine? The answer is that the child is likely to have periods of exacerbation and periods of remission. About one-third of children with migraine seem to have a spontaneous remission that can last 10 years or more. Boys seem to have a more favourable outcome. In essence, boys grow out of migraine but girls grow into it, often worsening during the perimenopause. Migraine typically ceases in later life in both sexes.

4

Case study

'It took me about 3–4 years to realize that I was having migraines. I was about 15 and had a really bad one and the doctor was called out because I was so ill. Up to that time my mother wasn't certain it was migraine. That severe attack lasted for about 5 days. From then on, I realized I was a migraine sufferer.

'The best time that I had was during my twenties and I only had occasional migraines then. There was no regular pattern at all. I'd probably go several months between attacks and that seemed to last most of my twenties. When I was going through a bad patch I was having migraines every 8–10 days lasting 2 days at a time. I've been on HRT now for several months and I only get a migraine attack once a month at the moment.'

Other types of migraine

Migraine aura without headache

Patients who have attacks of migraine with aura may lose the headache or the headache may become less of a feature. The headache may be minimal, often only noticed on bending down or shaking the head, or completely absent. A diagnosis should only be made if the patient has an established history of migraine with aura. Migraine aura without headache presenting *de novo* may require further investigation. It is rare for attacks to have always been without headache and if the onset of the first aura is after the age of 40, thromboembolic causes should be excluded.

Status migrainosus

Attacks of migraine may last longer than the generally accepted 72 h and, if prolonged, are sometimes termed 'status migrainosus'. However, this is a label rather than a diagnosis in itself. In practice, prolonged attacks are often due to the development of accompanying severe muscle contraction in neck and scalp muscles. The history reveals a typical migraine lasting up to 3 days followed by headache associated with tenderness in the scalp and neck muscles but with only mild nausea or photophobia. 'Status migrainosus' can also arise from medication misuse. A careful drug history will reveal over-frequent use of acute medication in preceding months.

Rare types of migraine

Other variants are listed below but the link of some of these with migraine is controversial. Further, the terms are often incorrectly used. In their true guise, they are rare and unlikely to be encountered in general practice. The referral of suspected cases to a neurologist or specialist clinic is advised.

Basilar migraine

Many of the symptoms of basilar migraine are more commonly associated with anxiety and attacks of hyperventilation. The symptoms clearly originate from the brainstem and include dysarthria, vertigo, tinnitus, diplopia and ataxia, in addition to the more typical aura symptoms. Visual symptoms usually appear first and amblyopia is not uncommon. This is followed by unsteadiness of gait and dysarthria. Tingling and numbness are noticed circumorally as well as in both hands and feet, spreading proximally to the wrists and ankles. These symptoms last from 10 to 45 min prior to the onset of the headache. Severe attacks may be associated with fainting and sudden loss of consciousness.

Hemiplegic migraine

Hemiplegic migraine begins in childhood, often precipitated by a minor head injury. Attacks cease during adolescence. Attacks of migraine with aura are associated with hemiplegia. The hemiplegia can persist for days or weeks. Altered consciousness, and sometimes coma, can occur. Headache is a variable feature of attacks and may be absent. In subsequent attacks, the opposite side may be affected. There is a family history of identical attacks in cases of familial hemiplegic migraine. This condition has been linked to a genetic defect in chromosome 19. Differential diagnosis includes stroke, focal seizures, and the rare cerebral autosomal dominant arteriopathy with subcortical infarcts and leukoencephalopathy (CADASIL)—also linked to chromosome 19.

Ophthalmoplegic migraine

The headache is associated with unilateral paresis of one or more of the cranial nerves III, IV and VI in the absence of underlying pathology. Symptoms may persist for over a week. There may be several months' remission before another identical attack, although the opposite side may be affected.

Retinal migraine

These are attacks of fully reversible monocular scotoma or blindness lasting less than 1 h with an associated headache. Ophthalmoscopic examination is normal between attacks.

Migrainous infarction

Permanent sequelae have rarely been reported following attacks of migraine. The most common lesions are visual, ranging from scotomas to field loss. It is difficult to establish a direct causal link as arterial degenerative disease and other risk factors can coexist with migraine. A diagnosis of migrainous infarction should only be considered if cerebral infarction occurs during the course of a typical migraine attack and other causes are excluded.

References

1 Headache Classification Committee of the International Headache Society. Classification and diagnostic criteria for headache disorders, cranial neuralgias and facial pain. *Cephalalgia* 1988; 8 (Suppl. 7): 1–96.
2 Blau JN. Migraine prodromes separated from the aura: complete migraine. *BMJ* 1980; 281: 658–60.
3 Russell MB, Olesen J. A nosographic analysis of the migraine aura in a general population. *Brain* 1996; 119: 355–61.
4 Blau JN. Classical migraine: symptoms between visual aura and headache onset. *Lancet* 1992; 340: 355–6.
5 Blau JN. Resolution of migraine attacks: sleep and recovery phase. *J Neurol Neurosurg Psychiatry* 1982; 45: 223–6.
6 Blau JN. Migraine postdromes: symptoms after attacks. *Cephalalgia* 1991; 11: 229–31.

CHAPTER 5

The Pathogenesis of Migraine

Numerous theories abound about the pathophysiology of migraine but the true nature of the condition remains a mystery. The difficulty with developing theories is that they have to account for the initiation of the attacks and all the symptoms: prodromes, aura, headache and associated symptoms, resolution and recovery. To date, no theory adequately explains the entire migraine process. The problem with studying patients with migraine is that they are otherwise fit and well. In addition, the episodic nature of migraine attacks and the need for most patients to retire to bed until the attack is over, make it is easy to understand the logistical problems of studying migraineurs. But the future is bright. Migraine research has never been more prolific than in recent years and this pace looks set to continue far into the next century. Newer imaging techniques are becoming increasingly less invasive, although the problem remains of getting the patient to the machine during an attack.

The vascular hypothesis

The most simplistic theory is the 'vascular hypothesis'. This had been considered by Thomas Willis (Fig. 5.1) as far back as the 17th century but was more formally proposed by Harold Wolff, Professor of Neurology in New York in 1938 (Fig. 5.2). The theory states that the visual symptoms of migraine aura are associated with intracerebral arterial vasoconstriction affecting the visual cortex in the occipital lobe. Wolff and coworkers found that progression of the aura could be arrested by inhalation of vasodilator agents such as amyl nitrate but this has not been replicated by other researchers. Conversely, headache was considered to be due to a reactive extracerebral vasodilatation which stretched nerve endings in the vessel wall. Nerve impulses relayed to the higher parts of the brain are perceived as headache. This mechanism of reactive hyperaemia is supported by the throbbing nature of the pain and its response to vasoconstrictors such as ergotamine.

The neural hypothesis

The vascular theory had strong support for many years. However, an

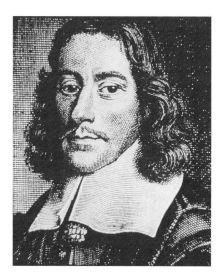

Fig. 5.1 Thomas Willis: the first person to propose the vascular theory. Courtesy of Dr J. Edmeads.

alternative hypothesis, that migraine is primarily a disturbance of brain function, was brewing. In 1941 Lashley, a physiologist who himself had migraine, noted that his visual aura travelled across his field of vision at a rate of 3 mm/min [1]. This was calculated on the basis that his aura usually lasted 20 min and the visual cortex is about 60 mm in

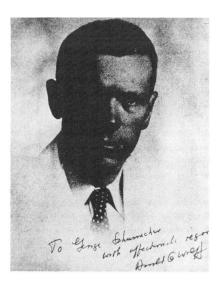

Fig. 5.2 Harold Wolff: the first person to conduct laboratory studies on headache. Courtesy of Dr J. Edmeads.

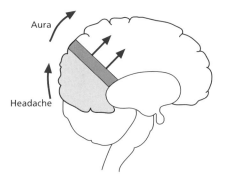

Fig. 5.3 Spreading depression in migraine.

length. His explanation for the aura was that a wave of intense excitation, propagated at a rate of 3 mm/min, moved across the visual cortex. This was followed by a wave of complete inhibition of activity, with recovery progressing at the same rate. Further credence for this theory came in 1944 when a Brazilian neurophysiologist working in Boston, Aristides Leão, published his observations on a process of neural activity which he termed 'spreading depression' [2]. Leão noted that this wave of reduced electrical activity elicited by a noxious stimulation advanced across the cerebral cortex of anaesthetized rabbits, pigeons and cats. Leão further noted that the wave of reduced electrical activity was associated with a simultaneous wave of marked dilation and increased blood flow in the pial arteries and veins, apparently as a secondary response to the neural changes [3]. These events were originally postulated as a possible explanation for tonic–clonic seizure pattern of experimental epilepsy. Together with Morrison, Leão raised the possibility that spreading depression may occur in migraine, noting that 'the marked dilatation of major blood vessels and the slow march of scotomas in the visual or somatic sensory sphere is suggestively similar to the experimental phenomena here described' [4] (Fig. 5.3).

In 1958 a Canadian, P.M. Milner, also commented on a possible link between migraine aura and Leão's spreading depression but the theory did not really gain ground until the work of Olesen and coworkers in Denmark during the 1980s. Their blood flow studies found reduced cerebral blood flow during the aura which developed before and outlasted the focal symptoms (Fig. 5.4) [5]. These studies suggest that, in migraine with aura, a spreading oligaemia moves across the cortex at a rate of 2–3 mm/min—similar to the rate described by Lashley—reportedly preceded by a phase of focal hyperaemia. The explanation for these vascular changes was that they occurred in response to a disturbance of brain function, or cortical spreading depression. It was considered that

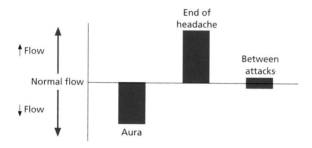

Fig. 5.4 Cerebral blood flow changes in occipital lobe.

5

cortical spreading depression was the underlying cause of the symptoms, i.e. cerebral blood flow changes in migraine may be an epiphenomenon.

But it is difficult to reconcile these events with the clinical symptoms of aura—particularly since aura symptoms are not identical. For example, they do not always last a finite 20 min, and may not always follow the pattern of scotomas and fortification spectra marching across the visual field. Then there is the additional problem of explaining sensory symptoms that often start in the hand and spread up the arm to the face. Further, positron emission tomography (PET) of a patient without aura also showed reduced blood flow during a spontaneous migraine headache [6]. Therefore the vascular theory that aura is associated with vasoconstriction and headache is associated with vasodilatation does not hold. But neither can neural changes account for the clinical symptoms of migraine, as 'spreading depression' affects a larger area than the isolated parts of the brain associated with aura symptoms. Evidence for spreading depression in humans is also very limited. To date, only one research group, using magnetoencephalography, have reportedly shown similar changes in humans to those seen in Leão's stimulated anaesthetized rabbits. Even if spreading depression is important in migraine, it still does not account for prodromal symptoms. Neither does it explain the headache, as the brain itself does not contain any pain receptors.

Trigeminovascular theory

Not surprisingly a combined theory has been developed to answer some of these issues. There is considerable evidence that the head pain of migraine is mediated by the trigeminovascular system. The trigeminovascular nerve is the main sensory nerve in the head, channelling orthodromic nociceptive impulses from blood vessels or other

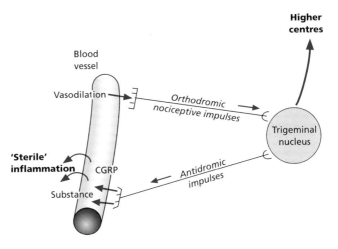

Fig. 5.5 Neurogenic inflammation.

pain-sensitive intracranial structures through to the higher centres of the central nervous system which register the impulses as pain.

During the 1980s Moskowitz, in Boston, proposed the theory of 'neurogenic' or 'sterile' inflammation (Fig. 5.5). Stimulation of the trigeminal nerve causes impulses travel the wrong way, antidromically, down the trigeminal axon from the cortex or other higher centres in the central nervous system to the cranial blood vessels. This triggers the secretion of neurotransmitters such as substance P and calcitonin gene-related peptide (CGRP). CGRP is a powerful vasodilator of cerebral arteries. Levels of CGRP are known to rise following stimulation of the trigeminal ganglion. Goadsby and Edvinsson have recently shown that this peptide is elevated during the headache phase of migraine and therefore may provide a possible marker for activation of the trigeminovascular system in migraine.

According to Moskowitz, the secreted transmitters combine with receptors in the vessel wall causing them to dilate and become leaky—the so-called neurogenic inflammation. In turn, pain impulses pass in the usual orthodromic route back to the brain stem and are interpreted as pain. This theory fitted nicely with the role of serotonin, or 5-hydroxytryptamine (5HT), in migraine since presynaptic 5HT1D receptors are located at both ends of the trigeminal axon. Serotonin has been shown to inhibit the release of substance P and CGRP, preventing the pain cycle. Thus, in Moskowitz's model, drugs such as ergotamine and the 'triptans' which act on 5HT receptors are effective in controlling pain by their inhibition of neurogenic inflammation. Unfortunately, the relevance of this model to the human situation is debatable, particularly since some drugs shown to be effective in migraine do not inhibit neurogenic inflammation and vice versa.

The role of 5-hydroxytryptamine (serotonin)

While debate about the mechanisms of migraine continues, the role of the neurotransmitter 5HT is unquestionable. 5HT is found throughout the body, mostly in the gut (90%) and blood platelets (8–10%), although a small amount is in the brain (1–2%). In the vascular system, 5HT can cause vasoconstriction or vasodilatation depending on the pre-existing vessel tone. It also promotes platelet aggregation.

The distribution of 5HT in the central nervous system forms a diffuse network. The midline raphe nuclei contain the nerve cell bodies of the major 5HT neurones. Pathways ascend to the basal ganglia, hypothalamus, limbic system and the cerebral cortex. Lance and his colleagues have found that in animal models, stimulation of the serotonergic brainstem raphe nuclei affects pathways projecting up to the cerebral cortex and can produce a 20% increase or decrease in cerebral blood flow. It is also involved in pain transmission as pathways from the same nuclei project downwards to a 'pain gating' system in the spinal cord.

Central 5HT mechanisms are also important in the hypothalamic control of mood and behaviour, motor activity, feeding and hunger, thermoregulation, sleep, certain hallucinatory states and possibly some neuro-endocrine control mechanisms.

5-hydroxytryptamine in migraine

Many factors implicate the importance of 5HT in migraine [7]. A 5HT releasing factor is present in the plasma during the headache phase of migraine and 5HT is released from its storage sites. Thus, 5HT levels in the bloodstream initially increase, followed by a decrease soon after the attack begins. 5-hydroxyindoleacetic acid (5HIAA), a metabolite of 5HT, is excreted in the urine in increasing amounts as the 5HT content of platelets falls. Central actions of 5HT can cause vascular changes, as well as influencing the endogenous pain control mechanisms that modulate the perception of pain from cranial vessels.

Pharmacological evidence shows that an injection of reserpine, which releases 5HT from body stores, induces migraine headache in susceptible subjects but not in normal controls. A migraine attack can be aborted by an intravenous infusion of 0.1% 5HT but its clinical use is limited by side-effects, include dyspnoea, chest tightness, nausea and

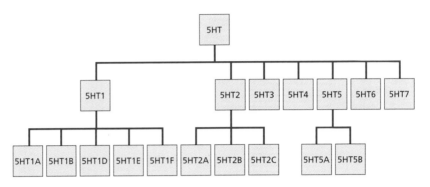

Fig. 5.6 5HT receptors.

generalized vasoconstriction resulting in faintness and paraesthesia. This has led to the development of specific migraine drugs acting on the 5HT system.

5-hydroxytryptamine receptors and migraine therapy

Gaddum and Picarelli were the first to propose the D (dibenzyline–phenoxybenzamine-sensitive) and M (morphine-sensitive) receptor classification for 5HT based on the differential sensitivity of 5HT-induced guinea-pig ileum contraction to some drugs. With the rapid advances in research, the existence of multiple 5HT receptors has been confirmed, necessitating the development of a structured system of nomenclature (Fig. 5.6) [8]. This is based upon the actions of specific and selective 5HT-receptor agonist and antagonists. The different receptor types in humans have been divided into four main groups: 5HT1, 5HT2, 5HT3, and 5HT4. 5HT1 receptors can be divided into five subtypes: 5HT1A, 5HT1B, 5HT1D, 5HT1E and 5HT1F. There are three subtypes of 5HT2 receptors: 5HT2A, 5HT2B and 5HT2C. Four additional recombinant receptors (5ht5A, 5ht5B, 5ht6 and 5ht7) provide strong evidence for the existence of three additional receptor classes, which will undoubtedly be fully classified in the near future.

The 5HT2B receptors have recently been suggested to play a crucial role in the initiation of migraine attacks. This may account for the efficacy of the prophylactic drugs, many of which act on these receptors: **Methysergide** is a 5HT2 receptor antagonist. It also has weak and non-selective 5HT1 receptor antagonist and partial agonist actions. **Pizotifen** is a 5HT1C and 5HT2 receptor antagonist.

Anti-nauseant drugs used in migraine, such as **metoclopramide**, act at 5HT3 receptors.

Drugs used in the acute treatment of migraine act on 5HT receptors: **ergotamine** is a partial agonist at 5HT2 but also acts on 5HT1D receptors. However, it is a non-selective drug with activity at α-adrenoceptors. It also has a narrow therapeutic window with unpleasant side-effects at high doses.

In view of the effectiveness of 5HT, it was argued that a drug could be developed which had the beneficial effect of aborting the migraine headache but with a lower side-effect profile. Research into the receptors relevant to migraine led to the production of **sumatriptan.** This drug acts as an agonist of 5HT1B receptors in the vasculature and 5HT1D receptors in nervous tissue. 5HT1B receptors are found both pre- and postsynaptically in the peripheral and central nervous systems. 5HT1D receptors are the most common type of 5HT-receptor subtype in the human brain. The 5HT1D receptor also functions as an 'autoreceptor' which controls the release of 5HT and other neurotransmitters. Sumatriptan does not readily cross the blood–brain barrier and its most likely mechanism of action in migraine is the selective cranial vaso-constriction, probably of the large cerebral arteries and the meningeal vasculature. However, sumatriptan also acts to inhibit the release of the neuropeptide CGRP from trigeminal nerve endings by activation of presynaptic 5HT1D receptors located on sensory nerve terminals. The administration of sumatriptan results in a reduction in the levels of CGRP at the same time as the headache is ameliorated.

More recent advances have been made with the newer 'triptans', **almotriptan, eletriptan, frovatriptan, naratriptan, rizatriptan** and **zolmitriptan**. In addition to the peripheral actions of sumatriptan on the trigeminovascular system, most of these drugs have central activ-ity within the brainstem. How relevant this is clinically remains un-certain at present as it would appear that the blood–brain barrier may not be normal during the headache of migraine allowing drugs with peripheral actions, such as sumatriptan, access to central sites. This concept is particularly important as new research suggests that vaso-constriction is not the principal mechanism of the triptans in pain re-lief. Further research will perhaps reveal the true mechanism of migraine therapies.

Other theories

Catecholamine levels rise and fall in plasma and these fluctuations have been shown to parallel the changes in plasma serotonin. Serum dopamine-β-hydroxylase, a marker of sympathetic activity, increases during migraine headache and vanillylmandelic acid (VMA), a catabolite of catecholamines, is excreted in increased amounts. The plasma level of noradrenaline (but not adrenaline) then declines. Although noradrenaline activates platelet-activating factor (PAF) and an infusion causes constriction of extracranial vessels, there is no clinical or experimental evidence to implicate catecholamines in the pathogenesis of migraine.

Histamine induces a generalized vasodilatation and elevated levels of histamine in migraineurs have been reported. It is thought that histamine may contribute to the vascular component of migraine arising from extracranial tissues.

Magnesium is known to influence vascular tone. Deficiency of magnesium induces platelet hyperaggregation and the release of central neurotransmitters in experimental subjects. Low brain levels of magnesium have been reported in migraine. Reports of magnesium as an acute migraine therapy have been promising.

Melatonin levels in the plasma have been shown to be reduced in migraineurs. It has long been recognized that migraine is linked to circadian rhythms, with most attacks beginning between the hours of 6 AM and 10 AM. Some trials with melatonin altering the sleep/wake cycles have shown some success in migraine therapy. Although melatonin is available without a prescription in some countries (not the UK), the long-term effects of melatonin used therapeutically are unknown.

Tyramine is a vasoactive amine that has been implicated in the pathogenesis of dietary migraine. It is present in several migraine triggers including cheese, other dairy products and some wines. Chocolate has little or no tyramine but does contain another vasoactive amine, β-phenylethylamine. Although early research suggested a promising link, recent studies have failed to provide definitive evidence that an abnormality of tyramine metabolism exists in migraine. Further, in the majority of migraineurs the link between ingestion of foods containing tyramine before the headache phase may be more related to prodromal cravings than to a triggering mechanism.

Platelets contain more than 90% of the serotonin in the body and this has given rise to the hypothesis that migraine is primarily a disorder of platelets, resulting in episodic platelet aggregation and 5HT release. There is evidence of platelet aggregation and a platelet-release reaction in migraine. The monoamine oxidase (MAO) activity of platelets is reported to be lower than that of control subjects. There is some suggestion that platelet hyperaggregability may be associated with migraine aura. However, brainstem serotonin is the more likely candidate involved in the generation of migraine; platelet aggregation and serotonin release are probably secondary events.

Prostaglandin release may play a role in migraine as prostaglandin antagonists have been reported to be of benefit in the treatment of acute attacks. This mechanism may be particularly relevant to some menstrual attacks, particularly if associated with dysmenorrhoea or menorrhagia.

5

Nitric oxide was, until 1987, considered to be little more than an atmospheric pollutant. Since then, the biology of this tiny, short-lived messenger has been identified as having extensive effects throughout the body, depending on the tissues involved. No specific receptors have been identified. Instead, it diffuses freely across membranes. It has been proposed that nitric oxide is involved in the initiation of migraine attacks and in the maintenance of the attack [9]. Certainly, nitric oxide synthase inhibitors have been shown some promise in the acute treatment of migraine. Further, there is some evidence that at least some of the effects of the triptans may be associated with inhibition of nitric oxide synthase activity.

Explaining the unexplained

Research may have begun to account for the mechanisms underlying the aura and headache but they do not explain how an attack is initiated or the development of prodromal symptoms.

Recent identification of a site of activation in the brainstem in spontaneous migraine attacks has led to the concept of a migraine 'generator' [10]. It is proposed that an abnormality may lead to an imbalance in brainstem regulation of the normal control of cerebral blood vessels and pain.

A key site for prodromes is the hypothalamus, sometimes described as the 'master of the endocrine orchestra'. This area of the brain is involved in the generation of circadian rhythms. It responds to stimuli by producing complex behavioural and emotional reactions including effects on sleep, hunger, thirst and mood changes such as elation, depression and irritability. It is worth noting that these are all changes noted by patients during the prodrome of migraine.

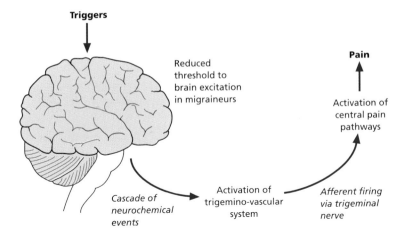

Fig. 5.7 Current concept of migraine mechanisms.

The future

Advances in migraine research are set to continue. The pathophysiology of migraine has become an exciting area with the potential for enormous therapeutic advances to be made. As research continues, it may become possible to link all the different pieces of the jigsaw together and uncover the elusive mechanism of migraine (Fig. 5.7).

References

1 Lashley KS. Patterns of cerebral integration indicated by the scotomas of migraine. *Arch Neurol Psychiatry* 1941; 46: 331–9.
2 Leão AAP. Spreading depression of activity in the cerebral cortex. *J Neurophysiol* 1944; 7: 359–90.
3 Leão AAP. Pial circulation and spreading depression of activity in the cerebral cortex. *J Neurophysiol* 1944; 7: 391–6.
4 Leão AAP, Morrison RS. Propagation of spreading cortical depression. *J Neurophysiol* 1945; 8: 33–45.
5 Olesen J, Friberg L, Olsen TS, Iversen HK, Lassen NA, Andersen AR, Karle A. Timing and topography of cerebral blood flow, aura and headache during migraine attacks. *Ann Neurol* 1990; 28: 791–8.
6 Woods RP, Iacoboni M, Mazziotta JC. Brief report: bilateral spreading cerebral hypoperfusion during spontaneous migraine headache. *N Engl J Med* 1994; 331: 1689–92.
7 Silberstein SD. Review. Serotonin (5HT) and migraine. *Headache* 1994; 34: 408–17.
8 Hartig PR, Hoyer D, Humphrey PP, Martin GR. Alignment of receptor nomenclature with the human genome: classification of 5-HT1B and 5-HT1D receptor subtypes. *Trends Pharmacol Sci* 1996; 17 (3): 103–5.

9 Thomsen LL. Investigations into the role of nitric oxide and the large intracranial arteries in migraine headache. *Cephalalgia* 1997; 17: 873–95.

10 Weiller H, May A, Limmroth V *et al.* Brainstem activation in spontaneous human migraine attacks. *Nature Med* 1995; 1: 658–60.

5

CHAPTER 6

What Causes Migraine Attacks?

There is no single cause for migraine. Imagine a migraine 'threshold' that is determined by an individual's genetic makeup. This threshold is raised or lowered by external factors, as well as internal changes in the brain. Varying trigger factors combine and may reach the threshold, initiating a migraine attack. This explains why missing a meal, flickering sunlight or lack of sleep do not always trigger an attack. However, if either is combined with a period of stress at work or falling oestrogen levels during the menstrual cycle, an attack may ensue. The mechanism of prophylactic therapy may be to raise the migraine threshold.

Triggers are diverse and so it is not surprising that many doctors do not feel that there is much benefit to be gained by trigger avoidance. However, a motivated patient can identify and avoid relevant trigger factors thereby reducing attack frequency. Identifying specific triggers relevant to the individual patient can be time-consuming as no migraine trigger applies to every patient and even in the same patient, different combinations of triggers may be responsible for different attacks. Further, triggers often change over the years: strenuous exercise, missed meals and late nights are common triggers in the young but in later life sleep, neck and dental problems may predominate (Fig. 6.1).

Migraine triggers (Table 6.1)

Triggers for migraine are no different from the factors that provoke 'nor-

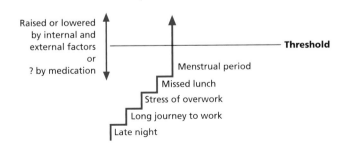

Fig. 6.1 The 'threshold' theory of migraine. Reproduced with permission from MacGregor EA. "Menstrual" migraine: towards a definition. *Cephalalgia* 1996; 16: 11–21.

Table 6.1 Migraine triggers.

Insufficient food
Specific foods
Sleep
Head and neck pain
Emotional triggers
Environment (weather/light/strong smells)
Hormonal changes
Illness

mal' headaches in apparently non-migrainous individuals. In some cases it may be difficult to distinguish triggers from prodromal symptoms. For example, someone who is photophobic in the prodromal stage will be more aware of sunlight flickering through the trees while driving. Similarly, prodromal carbohydrate cravings provoke a desire for chocolate. In both cases, the suspect trigger is more likely to be an early migraine symptom.

Insufficient food

Delayed or missed meals resulting in low blood sugar are probably the commonest migraine trigger [1]. This is particularly the case in children whose metabolic demands from growth and activity are not adequately met. But insufficient food may also be an important cause in adults. Missing breakfast typically triggers attacks late morning; missed lunch may trigger attacks late afternoon. If attacks are present on waking it is worthwhile considering the time of the evening meal—often very early. An easily digestible late night snack could be the answer.

Case study

Amanda is 45 and has a high-powered job as a civil servant. She has had migraine since her teens but recently attacks have been more frequent and she now has one every week. They last a couple of days but are worse on the first day. She has to go to bed with severe headache, nausea and vomiting. By the second day, the symptoms have eased off sufficiently that she can struggle in to work. She is worried about losing her job. She has not found any medication that will control the symptoms and is concerned that side-effects of prophylactic medication might impair her work. Besides, she does not like the idea of taking drugs every day and is interested in finding the cause of attacks. After keeping a daily diary of potential triggers for several weeks, she

Table 6.2 Some foods cited as triggering migraine.

Animal protein	Fish
Apples	Hot dogs
Bananas	Milk
Beans	Monosodium glutamate
Cereals	Nuts
Cheese	Onion
Chocolate	Rice
Citrus fruits	Shellfish
Coffee	Tomatoes
Egg	Wine

notices that she is often too busy to eat breakfast and rarely eats lunch during the working day. After a few weeks of eating breakfast and making time for snacks during the day, migraine frequency reduces to once every 4–6 weeks and symptoms respond better to medication.

Diet (Table 6.2)

Too many people strictly avoid suspect foods without first discovering whether or not they really contribute to their headaches. Moreover, craving for sweet foods such as chocolate is more typically a prodromal symptom, heralding the headache, rather than a trigger. Other triggers, such as perimenstrual hormone fluctuations and stress, may themselves be associated with sweet cravings.

Despite the more likely association between cravings and prodromal symptoms of migraine, food allergy is popularly considered as a migraine trigger. The most frequently cited culprits are red wine, cheese, citrus fruits and chocolate. But the word 'allergy' should not be used in relation to migraine as a true allergic response to an 'antigen' (in this case a suspect food) is associated with the production of specific measurable 'antibodies' in the body [2]. Despite intense research, no specific antigen–antibody reaction has been identified in migraine. It is therefore unlikely that allergy testing is worthwhile in migraine except in a minority of cases.

Skin-prick test or radioallergoabsorbent (RAST) testing is rarely indicated except for patients who develop rapid onset of symptoms in response to a specific food. Unfortunately, too many unqualified practitioners have offered unscientific tests, the results of which have led many migraineurs to follow strict diets which can cause nutritional problems if continued for long periods of time.

The term food 'sensitivity' or food 'intolerance' is used when symptoms are precipitated by non-immunological mechanisms. The usual presentation is chronic, rather than episodic, headache associated with chronic diarrhoea, pain, flatulence and bloating.

Rather than specific food intolerance, migraine could be triggered by vasoactive amines, particularly tyramine, histamine and phenylethylamine, found in foods such as cheese and chocolate [3]. Although research during the 1970s provided compelling evidence, it is clear that the true association between amines and migraine is not as clear as was first thought [4]. Even the popular theory of triggering migraine by eating chocolate does not stand up to more stringent research methods [5].

However, some food triggers do have scientific support. It is true to say that certain alcoholic drinks may trigger attacks in some susceptible individuals. Limited research does suggest that some alcoholic beverages contain chemicals that may directly affect blood vessels or provoke the release of other chemicals thought to initiate migraine attacks [6]. In this respect, the patient is sensitive to certain components of the alcoholic drink, particularly flavenoids. Drinks containing higher levels of flavenoids, such as certain red wines, are more likely to trigger attacks than pure drinks such as vodka.

Caffeine withdrawal has also been implicated as a migraine trigger. This is particularly the case for those patients who have a high intake of caffeine during the working week. A reduction in their intake, typically at weekends, may provoke attacks [7,8]. Although this has been associated with an increase in weekend migraine, other factors are also likely to provoke attacks at this time, particularly sleeping in, delayed breakfast and relaxation after the stress of the working week.

With all these factors in mind, it is obvious that the role of food triggers in migraine is complex. In practice, most migraineurs can eat whatever they like, as long as they eat enough to meet their energy demands. However, a few susceptible individuals have established a definite and reproducible time relationship between the consumption of certain foods, particularly alcohol, and the onset of migraine. Even in these patients, the suspect item may not trigger an attack on every occasion; patients frequently report that when they are feeling vulnerable to an attack an alcoholic beverage can tip the balance. If a patient suspects that a particular food does trigger an attack, that food should be avoided for a few weeks before it is reintroduced. If a large number of foods are involved, the patient should be referred to a dietician as elimination diets run the risk of causing malnutrition if they are not adequately supervised. Even this is likely to have limited success, as the diets are so restrictive that many people cannot maintain them, even within a clinical trial setting. In one study, 40% of patients had dropped out within the first 6 weeks and by the end of the study only 10% had improved, with a similar number unchanged or worse [9].

Dietary control can be sociably disabling—it is very difficult to avoid the chocolate mousse or French cheeses served with delicious wines at a dinner party. This can lead to fear of the possible effects of the food, which may in itself be sufficient to trigger an attack.

Exercise

Strenuous exercise in an unfit person can precipitate an attack. This puts many people off taking exercise when in fact regular exercise can help prevent migraine attacks. This is because it improves blood sugar balance, helps breathing, stimulates the body to release endorphins and encephalins and promotes a general sense of well being. Children appear to be particularly susceptible to the effects of strenuous exercise, developing migraine during an enduring game of football or a cross-country run. In many cases, these attacks can be prevented with adequate nutrition and glucose tablets during exercise.

Case study

James is 16. He has had migraine since he was 8. He does not have attacks very often and is aware that his main trigger is just before exam time, which he can control by eating regularly and not studying too late into the night. Recently, he has been training for his school rugby team but finds that strenuous training is triggering migraine. He is worried that he will lose his place in the team. Most of his training sessions have been after school and he frequently misses lunch. He tries eating some sandwiches on his way to training. He tops this up with glucose tablets at half-time and makes sure he drinks plenty of fluids. He does not have any more problems with migraine and is aiming to make the County team.

Hormones

Many women find that they are far more susceptible to a migraine attack around the time of their menstrual period, and a small percentage have attacks exclusively associated with menstruation. Most women can be treated with standard migraine management strategies but a few with obvious hormonal triggers may benefit from specific intervention.

Use of combined oral contraception can exacerbate migraine for some women and improve it in others. Migraine with aura is a contraindication to use of the combined oral contraceptive pill but not to other methods that do not contain ethinyloestradiol.

The climacteric is associated with increased frequency of migraine, particularly menstrual migraine. Stabilizing hormone fluctuations using hormone replacement therapy may be indicated if other climacteric symptoms are present.

Mechanisms and management strategies of hormonal triggers are discussed in detail in Chapter 10.

Illness

Headache is common with systemic infection, but migraine can also occur. It is uncertain whether illness is a trigger in its own right or if it lowers the attack threshold making the individual more prone to the effects of other triggers. Certainly, migraine attacks are more likely to occur when the patient is under par with a cold or flu.

Musculoskeletal pain

Neck and back pain can result from specific injury but even simple muscle tension unassociated with underlying pathology can result in headache and trigger migraine. Symptoms are frequently aggravated by poor posture, particularly those sitting at a computer for most of the day, or regularly driving long distances. Physical causes require physical treatments, although it may be several months before any benefit is seen.

Sleep

The association between sleep and migraine is poorly understood. Patients often report migraine on waking or soon after. Conversely, sleep during an attack may resolve symptoms. Lack of sleep can result from depression, anxiety or menopausal hot flushes or delayed bedtime due to social events, work or study. In either situation, migraine may ensue after a few sleepless nights. Conversely, sleeping in for even just half an hour longer than usual, or lying in bed dozing, can result in migraine. This may be one cause for weekend migraine. The mechanism is not understood. Sleep clearly plays an important role in migraine as during an attack patients comment that sleep can frequently abort an attack. Therefore, migraineurs are advised to follow a routine sleep pattern where possible.

Stress

Anxiety and emotion play an important role in headache and migraine. Most migraineurs cope with stresses at the time but have attacks when they relax—probably the reason why migraine occurs more often at weekends. Stress often results in other triggers with missed meals, poor sleep and muscle tension. Although stress is often unavoidable, it is important to avoid creating additional triggers.

Temporomandibular joint dysfunction

6

Temporomandibular joint dysfunction can be associated with muscle tension in the temporalis muscles, giving rise to headache, often daily, but occasionally triggering migraine.

Patients noted to have a 'clicking' jaw, particularly if they grind their teeth at night or if their jaws lock, may warrant referral to an orthodontist if simple measures are ineffective. Avoid other triggers that provoke muscle tension such as chewing gum [10].

Case study

Joanne is 15 and complains of 'migraine' which started several weeks ago. She has symptoms of generalized pain in both temples on most days, worse in the afternoon. She has no associated symptoms and is otherwise fit and well. Initially, she took painkillers but stopped these after a week as they were not effective. Examination was unremarkable other than tenderness over both temporomandibular joints and temporalis muscles, but no associated dysfunction. A diagnosis of muscle contraction headache was made and she was asked to keep a diary of her symptoms. A week later, she returns to the surgery. Her diary cards confirm her previous story and add nothing to the clinical picture. However, the doctor notices that she is chewing gum. On questioning, she had started chewing gum just before she developed the headaches. She thought it might help her diet and so was chewing several packets a day. The headaches resolved when she cut out the chewing gum.

Travel

Migraine and headache have been linked to travel, particularly by air. It remains uncertain as to whether pressure changes in aircraft triggers migraine, particularly with improved cabin pressures in modern planes. But travel is associated with a host of other triggers: fatigue from preparation and the trip itself, stress, missed or delayed meals, noise, cramped quarters, dry air and dehydration. These factors are all relevant triggers in their own right. Most also apply to other forms of travel.

Weather

Hot dry winds such as the Swedish Föhn, the Mediterranean Meltemi and the Canadian Chinook have long been associated with headache and general irritability. Weather changes are often cited as a trigger for migraine although the data are conflicting. In the UK, a study in London found no evidence for an effect of weather on migraine [11], although a study in Scotland suggested that a rise in barometric pressure was associated with increased migraine frequency [12].

Weekends

Migraine is more likely to occur at a weekend, particularly in those who work from Monday to Friday. This pattern is most likely to arise from a combination of events—stress release, late nights, sleeping in and delayed breakfast. Caffeine withdrawal, following a reduced caffeine intake at weekends compared with the working week, has also been implicated [13].

Visual display units

Visual display units (VDUs) are often believed to trigger headache. Many people blame the flickering screen when it is more likely that the trigger is related to how the individual works at the screen. In addition to increased muscle tension in the head and neck, working at a computer for long periods is associated with reduced blink rate and dry, sore eyes. These problems can be minimized by looking into the distance at regular intervals, blinking regularly, and performing some simple and quick stretching exercises during breaks.

Other causes

There are many other precipitating factors for migraine attacks. These include bright sunlight, strong smells, smoky environments, dehydration, cinema and loud sounds.

References

1 Blau JN, Cumings JN. Method of precipitating and preventing some migraine attacks. *BMJ* 1966; 2: 1242–3.

2 Hunter JO. Food allergy and intolerance. *Prescribers' J* 1997; 37: 193–8.

3 Kohlenberg RJ. Tyramine sensitivity in dietary migraine: a critical review. *Headache* 1982; 22: 30–4.

4 Zeigler DK, Stewart R. Failure of tyramine to induce migraine. *Neurology* 1977; 27: 725–6.

5 Marcus DA, Scharff L, Turk D, Gourley LM. A double-blind provocative study of chocolate as a trigger of headache. *Cephalalgia* 1997; 17: 855–62.

6 Littlewood JT, Gibb C, Glover V, Sandler M, Davies PT, Rose FC. Red wine as a cause of migraine. *Lancet* 1988; 1: 558–9.

7 Couturier EG, Hering R, Steiner TJ. Weekend attacks in migraine patients: caused by caffeine withdrawal? *Cephalalgia* 1992; 12: 99–100.

8 van Dusseldorp M, Katan MB. Headache caused by caffeine withdrawal among moderate coffee drinkers switched from ordinary to decaffeinated coffee: a 12 week double-blind trial. *BMJ* 1984; 289: 1579–80.

9 McQueen J, Loblay RH, Swain AR, Anthony M, Lance JW. A controlled trial of dietary modification of migraine. In: *New Advances in Headache Research*. Clifford Rose F, ed. London, Smith-Gordon, 1989: 235–42.

10 Dimitroulis G. Temporomandibular disorders: a clinical update. *BMJ* 1998; 317: 190–4.

11 Wilkinson M, Woodrow J. Migraine and the weather. *Headache* 1979; 19: 375–8.

12 Cull RE. Barometric pressure and other factors in migraine. *Headache* 1981; 21: 102–4.

CHAPTER 7

Making the Diagnosis: is it Migraine?

The first step in diagnosing migraine is identifying the problem. Few patients consult specifically for headache, often including it in a list of other complaints, mentioning in passing, or just as the consultation is being brought to a close. It is no wonder that patients complain that their doctor does not take their headaches seriously. In these situations, it is best to pick up on the headache but ask the patient to make another appointment to discuss the problem. Providing a diary card on which to record symptoms before the next visit can be very useful for both patient and doctor.

There are numerous different types of headaches, which occur for numerous different reasons. If a headache is sufficiently troublesome that the person seeks medical help, doctors cannot provide the most effective treatment unless they know exactly which type of headache they are treating. For most other medical ailments, the suspected diagnosis can be confirmed with tests. But no diagnostic test can confirm the most common headaches such as migraine or tension-type headache. This means that the diagnosis is based essentially on the replies given by the patient to the questions posed by the doctor. The examination is essentially normal. It is not surprising that the diagnosis is not always easy.

The major fear among patients and doctors is that the headache is caused by a brain tumour. Fortunately, the pattern of migraine is so typical that, once recognized, it should rarely be confused with more sinister and rarer conditions. These are discussed in Chapter 13.

A common problem is when several headaches coexist, confusing both patient and doctor. In a study of patients with a diagnosis of migraine who were referred to a specialist migraine clinic, over a quarter had an additional headache to migraine [1]. Failure to recognize and manage the additional headache was the most common cause of treatment failure. Careful history-taking of each headache present can prevent this problem.

A suggested method for taking the history follows, but other methods have been tried and tested [2]. Each doctor must find the method that suits him or her. In a general practice setting, time is of the essence—not just to make the diagnosis, but to do so in such a way that the patient can be reassured. The following text outlines one approach. The number of questions listed and suggestions for examination may appear daunting and time consuming. However, not all questions are necessary and a flexible approach enables both history and examination to be adapted to each consultation given the problems of the patient and the time constraints of the doctor. The 6–10 min available in general practice in the UK may not be sufficient unless much of the history is already known from previous consultations. Extra time spent may prove to be cost effective—studies show that consultation time influences the degree of patient satisfaction, with fewer prescriptions at the end of the consultation and subsequent reduced consultation rate [3].

7

Diagnostic criteria

Many medical ailments have been subject to the development of diagnostic criteria—just think back to the endless lists learned at medical school. Hippocrates is said to be the first to have recognized that headaches could be classified into primary and secondary conditions. Primary headaches include migraine and tension-type headache. Secondary headaches arise secondary to other conditions such as hangover, head injury, meningitis, or sinusitis. This simple differentiation had a powerful effect on treatment of headache as primary conditions obviously require quite different management from secondary headaches—the latter responding best to treatment of the underlying primary condition. Over the centuries, the classification has become more complex and has included specific diagnostic criteria. The first diagnostic criteria for migraine were introduced in 1962 by the Ad Hoc Committee on Classification of Headache. These were refined in 1988 by the Headache Classification Committee of the International Headache Society, who published the paper 'Classification and diagnostic criteria for headache disorders, cranial neuralgias and facial pain' [4] (see Appendix E). This document aimed to help physicians establish a specific headache diagnosis, primarily for research purposes. Their use has enabled more structured and comparative research to be undertaken. Unfortunately, they have also slipped into more general use leading to the development of checklists for doctors as an aid to diagnosis. These may provide a useful tool for the busy GP but they have severe limitations. Although specific, the diagnostic criteria are not very sensitive, for example they will diagnose a simple hangover as a migraine. Neither do many patients have great confidence in the doctor who relies on diagnostic and management aids. More importantly, they will not help the GP pick up additional headaches that may be the true reason why the patient presents in the surgery.

There are several models for consultation in general practice, for example task-orientated, goal, problem-solving, each of which may be appropriated for different patients. These should be borne in mind when developing your own approach [5,6].

Diagnosis in clinical practice

In itself, taking a history of migraine is straightforward and a diagnosis can usually be made from the responses to a few essential questions are outlined below. All remaining questions are confirmatory or help to identify causes and assess potential management strategies. In practice it is not always so straightforward as many patients present because of the development of an additional headache which can cloud the picture unless you ask the right questions. Correct diagnosis of each headache is essential to effective management. It should be possible to cover the basic requirements within 10 min, otherwise ask the patient to return for a fuller assessment. The GP has the advantage that most of the answers to the general questions will already be known. Similarly, much of the suggested examination may have been performed on earlier occasions, although a few points are mandatory.

Taking a history

'Tell me about your headaches.' In an ideal world, patients should be allowed to tell their own story. Time constraints rarely make this feasible and it is necessary to ask a few pertinent questions to structure the consultation. Unless the patient is particularly verbose or several headaches coexist, the diagnosis can usually be made in a few minutes.

Essential diagnostic questions

'How many different headaches do you have?' is a useful opening question and can prevent confusion and time wasted.

Most patients can readily distinguish between different headaches as each type usually follows a typical pattern of onset, timing and symptoms. If the patient has only one headache, the consultation is likely to be straightforward. If two or more are present, it is necessary to take a separate history for each headache. In such cases migraine is often a

Table 7.1 Differential diagnosis: headache in adults.

Acute headache		Recurrent headache	
Common	Rare	Common	Rare
See Recurrent	Temporal arteritis	Muscle contraction	Cluster headache
Sinusitis	Meningitis	Migraine	Post-traumatic
Dental	Encephalitis	Emotional tension	Neuralgia
Head trauma	Subarachnoid	Dental	Temporal arteritis
	haemorrhage	Medication misuse	Intracranial pathology
	Tumour		
	Phaeochromocytoma		

7

long-standing condition but a more recent headache is the one of concern to the patient. Do not accept that the patient's diagnosis is correct, for example 'eye strain' or 'sinus' headaches which can be misleading when the true diagnosis may be migraine. Alternatively, the patient may label the headache as migraine when the true diagnosis is muscle contraction headache or even medication misuse (Table 7.1).

The following questions should be repeated for each identified headache. Typical responses for migraine are given. Responses for potential tumours and other headaches are discussed in Chapters 13 and 14.

Age at onset

'*How old were you when the headache started?*' This question highlights a recent or long-standing history. Recent headaches are of greater concern. Migraine typically starts in the young, sometimes in childhood but more typically in teens or early twenties. It rarely starts *de novo* after age 50, although it is not uncommon for migraine to return in later life after a period of respite.

Frequency of attacks

'*How often do you have attacks?*' The frequency of migraine varies throughout life but patients rarely seek help until attacks become more frequent or severe. Frequent headaches should raise questionmarks in the diagnosis. Daily, progressive headaches are cause for concern. It is unusual for migraine to occur more often than once a week and, even in these cases, the diagnosis should be questioned. Daily headaches are not migraine but migraine may be superimposed on daily headache. Any patient reporting 'daily migraines' needs to be asked how the pattern of symptoms has changed over time. Although pathology needs exclusion, it is more common that an additional muscle contraction or tension headache has developed. All medication taken should be recorded, as medication misuse can develop, exacerbating daily headache.

Duration of attacks

'*How long does an attack typically last if you don't take treatment, or if treatment is not effective?*' Most migraines will last part of a day, up to 3 days. Attacks are typically shorter in children—sometimes less than a couple of hours—but lengthen with advancing years.

Episodicity

'*How do you feel between attacks?*' The response is usually 'Fine'. Patients with continued symptoms between attacks may have more than one type of headache.

Symptoms

'*Describe a typical attack.*' If the diagnosis is migraine, the patient can describe some or all of the stages of a typical attack. Some patients can spontaneously recount symptoms, others need prompting along the following lines. The order will need to be varied according to the patient's response.

• '*What time of day do attacks typically start?*' Migraine is typically present on, or soon after, waking but do not often wake the patient from sleep. Peak time at onset is between 8 AM and 10 AM. Headache associated with medication misuse and raised intracranial pressure are characteristically worse on waking. Muscle contraction headache usually develops over the course of the day.

• '*Where do you get the pain?*' Patients will usually point to one side of the head, which may alternate between or during attacks. Although typically unilateral, bilateral headache does not discount migraine, occurring in about 30% of attacks. The headache can swap sides between and during attacks. Neck pain is also common before and during migraine, sometimes radiating to the shoulder. Migraine can be associated with an underlying muscle contraction headache which can increase the frequency of migraine attacks and requires specific treatment. A more generalized and unremitting 'pressure' headache is more typically associated with depression.

• '*Describe the pain.*' The headache of migraine is usually described as a throbbing, pounding headache. Sometimes a patient says that their

Table 7.2 Differential diagnosis: aura.

Migraine aura
Panic attacks
Hypoglycaemia
Transient ischaemic attack
Epilepsy
Arteriovenous malformation
Retinal detachment
Glaucoma
Demyelinating disease

7

head feels as if it will explode and are frightened that a blood vessel may burst during an attack.

- *'Does light, sound or smell bother you more than usual?'*; *'Do you feel sick, are you sick?'* During an attack hypersensitivity to the light, sound and smell is common. Light may also aggravate the headache. Nausea and, less often, vomiting are aggravated by movement. Despite this, some patients are hungry and feel the need to eat carbohydrates. Others cannot face food until the recovery stage.

- *'Do you notice any problems with your vision, or any tingling or numbness in any part of your body either before or during attacks?'*; *'Describe what happens'*; *'How long do these symptoms last?'* These questions identify the typical focal neurological symptoms of migraine aura and help to differentiate them from neurological symptoms requiring further evaluation. Bright scintillating scotomas lasting 20 min before onset of headache is a typical aura. These are often perceived by the patient as affecting only one eye but careful evaluation in future attacks confirms that both visual fields are affected. Gradual development of symptoms also distinguishes migraine aura from the sudden onset of sinister pathology (Table 7.2). Aura symptoms are discussed in more detail in Chapters 4 and 13. Dizziness, dysphasia, poor concentration, irritability and general malaise are common both before and during the headache and all improve with resolution of headache.

- *'Do you notice any earlier warning symptoms before the headache?'* Often prodromal symptoms are only identified once the patient knows what to look for. Friends and family may be more aware of subtle changes in mood or behaviour than the patient is. Prompting with direct questions can elicit unusual tiredness, elation or food cravings, which can help confirm the diagnosis.

- *'How do attacks end?'* Symptoms usually resolve slowly, with sleep, or with vomiting. Typical descriptions of the recovery stage include: 'hungover', 'washed-out', 'drained', 'relieved' and less commonly 'elated'.

Disability

• *'What do the headaches stop you from doing?'* Migraine can cause significant disability with time lost from work, household duties and leisure, particularly if attacks are severe and/or frequent. This has important implications for treatment as disabling attacks require more aggressive therapy than mild, infrequent attacks.

Additional questions

Treatment

• *'What do you do when you have a migraine?'* Patients should be encouraged to describe medication taken, as well as what they physically do—go to bed, lie still, sleep, etc. Those who continue working often state that they can only carry out limited tasks during at attack.
• *'What treatments have you tried in the past?'* Many treatments that appear to fail in migraine would succeed if taken in adequate doses, sufficiently early in attacks. Establish what has failed in the past, and why, before recommending treatments higher up the treatment ladder as first-line therapy. Patients with frequent headaches should be carefully questioned about drug use to exclude medication misuse.

Triggers

• *'Have you found any triggers for attacks?'* Most patients can list at least a couple of triggers spontaneously and will identify several more if prompted with a list. More information is given about triggers in Chapter 6.
• *'Is there any pattern to attacks?'* Patients may notice attacks occur more often at weekends or linked to menstruation, which can be managed accordingly.

General questions

Most of the following will already be known to the physician but confirm that there have been no recent changes to the patient's general health.

Systemic review

Most patients presenting purely with migraine are otherwise fit and well. Symptoms suggestive of systemic disease require more detailed questioning.

Past medical history

There is rarely a relevant medical history for migraine although some patients may time the onset subsequent to a head injury, illness or emotional upset. In most cases it is impossible to know if the event was truly the initiator of migraine. Travel sickness and recurrent abdominal pain in childhood have been linked to the development of migraine in later life but this association is not diagnostic. Comorbid conditions should be considered, particularly depression which may require specific management. Work difficulties, marital problems, alcoholism, etc. need consideration. Medical conditions relevant to therapy should be considered, for example peptic ulcer or uncontrolled hypertension would contraindicate non-steroidal anti-inflammatory drugs (NSAIDs) or triptans, respectively.

Drugs

Headache is listed as a side-effect of almost every available drug. However, some drugs have been particularly associated with increased headache. These include the combined oral contraceptive pill, although headaches usually resolve with continued use. Occasionally increased frequency and severity of headache or migraine may necessitate adjustments to treatment or even withdrawal. Frequent use of acute treatments can lead to daily medication misuse headache. Specific drugs, particularly vasodilators, prescribed for coexisting conditions, may worsen migraine. A careful drug history is necessary to ensure that there is no incompatibility between drugs used for migraine and those taken for other indications.

Social history

Alcohol sometimes triggers migraine but can relieve the headache of muscle tension. Several occupations can increase the likelihood of migraine. Stressful jobs create obvious triggers which can be specifically identified. A secretary working at a visual display unit (VDU) for several hours at a stretch will develop muscle tension unless she takes regular breaks. Shift work can disrupt sleep and dietary routines. Unemployment and redundancy carry the risk of depression. Personal or family problems may be relevant.

The impact of headache on the patient's life should be discussed. It is not uncommon for patients to fear making arrangements in case they are disrupted by a migraine. This cycle of fear can be broken with effective management but may require additional psychological treatment.

Family history

A family history may be present but is not necessary to confirm the diagnosis. A family history of arterial disease may be relevant if vasoconstrictor drugs are considered.

And finally

End the history with a question such as: *'Is there anything else you want to mention before I examine you?'*; *'Why have you come to see me now?'*; *'What worries you about your headaches?'*; or even *'Lots of people when they get bad headaches think they may have something nasty like a brain tumour. What about you?'* Many patients have fears which they find hard to express. A simple question can prevent the patient leaving the consulting room still harbouring fear of a brain tumour that they have been frightened to ask about. The latter question has the advantage of enabling the doctor to know what the patient's ideas are so that they can be reinforced or refuted, and developed into management plans. This can help forge a better bond between doctor and patient. Patients often do not give an immediate answer to the question, but wait until they are being examined. This may be because they feel less vulnerable during a non-threatening examination. Eye contact is lost and the break in tension may permit the patient to release information or ask questions that are important.

Examination

Migraine is diagnosed by taking a careful history, but a physical examination should not be omitted, especially at the first presentation. The main purpose of the examination is to reassure patients. Patients and their family are often worried that there is a serious cause for the headaches such a brain tumour or stroke. Patients expect a physical examination and may be less likely to agree with the doctor's perspective and subsequent management recommendations if this is not done. The examination can be brief, but should be thorough [7]. In patients seen in a specialist clinic, fewer than 1% have headaches secondary to intracranial disease, and all have signs of it. The mental state will have been assessed while taking the history. Pulse, blood pressure and auscultation for cardiac abnormalities and bruits should be checked first and are particularly important if vasoconstrictor drugs such as ergotamine or the triptans are considered. Examining the jaw can identify temporomandibular joint dysfunction that can give rise to headache. Examination of the neck and cervical spine may reveal muscle contraction, cervical spondylosis or even meningism.

A rapid neurological examination

It is unnecessary to check every aspect of neurological function and a routine screen should take no more than 5 min. Particular attention should be paid to examination of the cranial nerves, tendon reflexes and optic discs. If the history suggests that there is a more sinister cause for the headache, a full neurological appraisal is necessary. It is of great comfort to patients when doctors explain that the findings are 'normal' and that this is to be expected in migraine. **When time is short, a minimum examination should include blood pressure and examination of the optic fundi.** Details on how to obtain a video of a 3-min neurological examination for use in recurrent headaches are in Appendix A.

Entering the consulting room

You can assess a great deal about a patient when they walk through the door. You can diagnose Parkinson's disease by the shuffling gait and cogwheel rigidity on handshake. Cerebellar disease is associated with a broad gait. Patients with migraine presenting between attacks will have a normal gait and appear well. Mood is worth assessing as patients with depression can often present with headache.

While taking the history

Speech, mood and memory can be assessed by the patient's response to questions.

With the patient sitting

At the end of the history, request permission from the patient before the examination.
• First check **pulse** and **blood pressure** and assess for fever, taking the temperature if indicated.
• Examine the **cardiovascular** and **respiratory** systems.

- Auscultate the **carotids** and **orbits** for bruits. This may disclose a systolic bruit suggesting the presence of an aneurysm, angioma or stenosis of the vessels. Breath sounds can be obscured by asking the patient to hold his or her breath for a few seconds. Skull bruits are often heard in children under the age of 10 and are rarely of any pathological significance.
- Inspect the **spine**.
- Palpate the **superficial temporal arteries**. These may be tender after a recent attack of migraine. A hard, swollen and tender artery in a patient over 55 suggests temporal arteritis.
- Examine the **neck** for local muscle tenderness and limitation of lateral flexion. Exclude meningeal irritation.
- Examine the **jaw** for temporomandibular dysfunction by placing the fingers of each hand over the jaw joints and asking the patient to open and close his or her mouth.
- Check the temporal **visual fields** (cranial nerve II) by confrontation. While the patient is seated, raise both your arms so that your index fingers are at eye level and about 80° peripheral to each eye. Ask the patient to look straight at your nose and point to whichever finger you move. This will reveal homonymous hemianopia if the patient fails to notice movement on one side (cerebral hemisphere lesion) and sensory inattention if the patient only points to one side when you move both (parietal lobe lesion). If any defect is found using this technique, the nasal field must be checked.
- Examine the **fundi** (cranial nerve II) to exclude papilloedema or optic atrophy. Subhyaloid haemorrhages may be observed after subarachnoid bleeding.
- Examine the **pupils** (cranial nerves II and III) and their reactions. Progressive enlargement of a pupil may suggest compression of the third nerve and immediate action should be taken. The dilated pupil is always on the side of the expanding lesion. A small pupil associated with an ipsilateral slight ptosis suggests Horner's syndrome—a cervical sympathetic defect. Test the light reflex by shining a torch into each eye and ensuring that both pupils constrict equally—the direct and consensual responses.
- Assess **external ocular movements** (cranial nerves III, IV and VI). Ask the patient about diplopia. Check for nystagmus. Test accommodation. The sixth nerve has a long intracranial course and a bilateral palsy is seen in cerebral oedema or a unilateral palsy may be found on the side of a lateral sinus thrombosis. Impairment of adductive and vertical eye movements suggest a third nerve palsy, usually associated with ptosis as well as a ipsilateral fixed and dilated pupil.

7

- Check **facial movements**, asking the patient to open his or her mouth fully and keep it open (cranial nerve V) while you try to close it using the palm of one hand. Asking the patient to smile and raise his or her eyebrows (cranial nerve VII) can ensure that movements are symmetrical.
- Assess **hearing** (cranial nerve VIII) by rubbing your thumbs against your fingertips about 3 cm from the patient's ears. If any deafness is suspected, examine the ears with an auroscope and check Rinne and Weber tests.
- Check **palatal movements** (cranial nerve X) asking the patient to open his or her mouth and say 'aah' while examining the uvula with a torch to ensure that is remains central.
- Assess **sternomastoid and trapezius** (cranial nerve XI) by asking the patient to push against your hand which has been placed on the forehead. Weakness suggests dystrophia myotonica, polymyositis or myasthenia gravis. Beware of the patient with neck pain and cervical spondylosis who can also have weakness. Muscle tenderness is usually apparent in these cases.
- Examine the **tongue** (cranial nerve XII), asking the patient to stick his or her tongue out at you and waggle it from side to side. Observe for muscle wasting and fasciculation. In unilateral lesions the tongue deviates to the *normal* side at rest and to the *paralysed* side on protrusion. Lateral movement is slower in motor neurone disease or cerebrovascular disease, and is clumsy in cerebellar dysfunction.
- Examine the **arms**. Look for muscle wasting or fasciculation. Tone may have been assessed with a handshake. Ask the patient to put his or her arms out and pretend to play the piano. Pyramidal tract lesions affecting motor function will result in slow and clumsy movements on the affected side. Ask the patient to turn the hands so that the palms face down, and close his or her eyes. Pyramidal dysfunction causes the arm on the affected side to gradually pronate and drift downwards. Check biceps and triceps tendon reflexes.
- Check **finger–nose** test for coordination.
- Check **sensation** by stroking the skin on the backs and palms of the hands, asking the patient whether it feels the same on both sides.

With the patient lying down

- Examine the **abdomen** if indicated.
- Examine the **legs** for muscle wasting, tone, and fasciculation. Check knee and ankle tendon reflexes. Perform **heel–shin** test for coordination.

- Check **sensation** by gently stroking skin on the back of each foot asking the whether it feels the same on both sides.
- Assess **plantar responses**.

With the patient standing

- Ask the patient to stand with the feet together, first with eyes open, then with eyes shut—**Romberg's test**. Cerebellar dysfunction will cause the patient to lose balance whether the eyes are open or closed. Joint position sense is defective if balance is only affected with the eyes closed, when visual feedback is lost.
- Check **heel–toe walking** to assess for cerebellar disease. Watch the patient **turn**—overbalancing is a sign of defective postural control.

Note that tests of smell (cranial nerve I), corneal response, facial sensation, jaw jerk (cranial nerve 5), and pharyngeal sensation (cranial nerve IX) have been omitted as they are rarely abnormal in isolation.

Investigations

Investigations do not contribute to the diagnosis of migraine; if you are sure of the diagnosis there is no need to investigate.

Some patients expect to have a scan. This provides little valuable information as there is only a 1 in 2000 chance of a positive finding. Further, few people are aware how unpleasant the experience is—it is not recommended for claustrophobic patients. Many patients request investigations for the reassurance that they do not have a brain tumour or other serious underlying pathology. This may be avoided if, on the basis of a sound history and examination, the doctor explains that everything is normal and that there is no indication for further investigation at this time.

Investigations are indicated if history and/or examination suggest that the headache may be secondary to underlying pathology. Examples indicating investigation or referral include: if there has been a recent change in the clinical features of the attacks that are not typical of migraine, in the presence of abnormal neurological signs, or if the onset of the first attack occurs over the age of 50. Beware of using investigations in order to reassure patients—false positive findings can cause harm. Although it may be necessary for a few who will not be reassured in the absence of a 'brain scan', others become more concerned believing that the doctor must think there is something seriously wrong if further tests need to be considered.

- **Full blood count and erythrocyte sedimentation rate** may detect the presence of infection or temporal arteritis.
- **Plain radiography** of the skull is normal in most patients with headache but may be indicated if there is a history of head injury or if symptoms/examination are suggestive of a tumour, particularly of the pituitary gland.
- **Lumbar puncture** confirms infection (meningitis or encephalitis). It should be used if subarachnoid haemorrhage is suspected and computed tomography (CT) scanning is either unavailable or the results are inconclusive—CT scans may be normal in 10–15% of all subarachnoid haemorrhage.
- **Electroencephalography (EEG)** is of little diagnostic value in migraine but may be considered if a clinical diagnosis suggests features of epilepsy, such as loss of consciousness occurring in association with migraine [8].
- **CT scanning** demonstrates structural lesions including tumour, vascular malformations, haemorrhage and hydrocephalus. If intracranial or subarachnoid haemorrhage is suspected, CT scan without contrast can detect recent bleeds—magnetic resonance imaging (MRI) may miss fresh blood. It may be necessary to give an intravenous injection of contrast material to highlight a suspected tumour or vascular lesion. Indications for CT scanning are persistent focal neurological deficits, symptoms or signs suggestive of an arteriovenous malformation and haemorrhagic stroke.
- **MRI** produces better definition of soft tissue abnormalities than CT scanning and is the investigation of choice for cerebral infarction. MRI with gadolinium is the investigation of choice for meningeal pathology. Although CT scanning can detect most tumours, MRI is more sensitive as it can detect infiltrating tumours and very small tumours which are only a few millimetres in diameter.
- **Cerebral angiography** is rarely required as a primary investigation and its use is limited by its invasiveness. If CT or MRI confirm arteriovenous malformation, angiography is used to define the extent of the lesion and demonstrate feeding and draining vessels.
- **Isotope scanning** and **Doppler flow studies** are only of value for research in migraine.

The attack diary card—a diagnostic tool

A headache diary can be an invaluable tool, particularly if the diagnosis is unclear or more than one type of headache is present. It can also be useful if medication misuse is suspected. Patients should be asked to keep a daily record of all their symptoms and all treatments taken for headache, including dose and time(s) taken. If the patient has migraine, a clear pattern of episodic headaches will be apparent with freedom from symptoms between attacks. Migraine attacks may also be evident as more severe headache with nausea on a background of daily headache. In the latter case, the migraine cannot effectively be managed until the daily headache is treated.

Conclusions: how to get it right

Making a diagnosis of migraine based on the suggested approach may appear time consuming. However, a primary care physician has the advantage of having treated a patient for several years and so, for many of the questions, the answers will already be known. Similarly, an extensive examination is unnecessary, although blood pressure and fundoscopy are mandatory. In most cases, the examination is more of a therapeutic than diagnostic measure. In cases of doubt about the diagnosis, diary cards are invaluable. The diagnosis should be reviewed at follow-up visits, particularly in cases of treatment failure. Always be on the lookout for coexisting headaches, which can confuse the picture.

Case study

Derek is a 36-year-old banker. He has had migraine since childhood but it was not a problem until he was involved in a car accident 2 years ago in which he says he injured his neck. He currently has two to three migraine attacks each month, typically at weekends. Attacks last most of one day and he is free from symptoms between attacks. He is aware of an imminent attack on waking but cannot describe any specific symptoms. Over the morning, pain starts in the back of the neck and the right shoulder. As the pain intensifies, it radiates into the right temple where it settles for the duration of the attack. He experiences mild nausea but never vomits. He is photophobic and phonophobic. Massage eases the localized muscle tenderness. He has to go to bed, and sleep can resolve most of the symptoms. He also gets 'normal' headaches if he works too long at his computer and when driving. These have become more frequent. He has found over-the-counter treatments effective in the past. These have stopped working and only take the edge off the pain so he no longer takes them. He is desperate to find some relief as the headaches are affecting his work.

Comment

It is not uncommon for an increase in migraine frequency to link to an increase in what patients describe as 'normal' headaches. The more severe symptoms are indicative of migraine without aura, possibly triggered by recent exacerbation of neck problems. Weekends often provide additional triggers of late nights, sleeping in, delayed or missed breakfast, and relaxation after stress. The first management approach is to provide effective acute therapy. Identification and avoidance of trigger factors might prove useful. Physical treatments would reduce the neck trigger. In Derek's case, a combination of an analgesic and antiemetic relieved the acute symptoms of migraine. He was interested in acupuncture and found that it reduced the frequency of his 'normal' headaches as well as the migraines.

7

Case study

Claire is 22 and is in her final year at university, studying English Literature. She states that she gets headaches a couple of times a month which do not bother her as she usually knows the cause and a couple of paracetamol make her better. However, she has been getting an increasing number of 'migraines' which she has had since she was 8. She used to only get them once or twice a year and they only lasted a day at the most. In the last couple of months she has had five or six attacks, each lasting a couple of days. Between attacks, she feels fine. They often start late morning or late afternoon when she is studying. She notices that she cannot see all the words on the page. This bright spot slowly gets bigger and develops a broken edge (she draws imaginary zigzags with her finger) which moves towards the edge of her vision before disappearing. The whole process lasts about 20 min from start to finish. She says that in some attacks they appear more in her right eye, in others in the left eye. In the last attack, she found that as the vision cleared she developed tingling in the fingers of her left hand which gradually spread up her arm into her face. This took about 10 min and then cleared. She was frightened by this as she had never experienced it before and thought she was having a stroke. Then she developed her usual throbbing headache and felt sick. She went to bed but pain and nausea prevented sleep. In a typical attack she would be sick and then she could sleep the rest of the attack off. She does not bother to take drugs because she feels too sick.

Comment

Claire describes migraine with aura. She has had migraine for 14 years which she self-treated effectively and so did not require medical advice. The reason she seeks help now is the increased frequency of attacks which she fears will affect her final exams and the development of new symptoms which she worries may be a stroke. Careful questioning revealed that her parents had recently divorced and she was also working several evenings a week as a waitress to pay back a bank loan. She was sleeping and eating badly. A thorough examination was normal but enabled the doctor to reassure her that her symptoms were migraine and not indicative of anything sinister. The doctor discussed the possible reasons behind the increased frequency of attacks such as exam worries, lack of sleep and poor diet, and suggests that she discuss some of her problems with her personal tutor at university.

7

References

1   Laughey WF, MacGregor EA, Wilkinson MIP. How many different headaches do you have? *Cephalalgia* 1993; 13: 136–7.
2   Blau JN. How to take a history of head or facial pain. *BMJ* 1982: 1249–51; 285.
3   Hughes D. Consultation length and outcome in two group general practices. *J R Coll Gen Pract* 1983; 33: 143–7.
4   Headache Classification Committee of the International Headache Society. Classification and diagnostic criteria for headache disorders, cranial neuralgias and facial pain. *Cephalalgia* 1988; 8 (Suppl. 7): 1–96.
5   Pendleton D. *Doctor–Patient Communication.* Academic Press, 1983.
6   Pendleton D, Schofield T, Tate P, Havelock P. *The Consultation—An Approach to Learning and Teaching.* Oxford, Oxford University Press, 1984.
7   Donaghy M. A basic neurological examination. In: *Neurology.* Donaghy M, ed. Oxford, Oxford University Press, 1997: 7–31.
8   Sand T. EEG in migraine: a review of the literature. *Funct Neurol* 1991; 6: 7–22.

CHAPTER 8

Management Strategies for Migraine

When the patient doesn't respond to the well known migraine treatments it is very important for the doctor to support the patient and keep trying. Patients need help. They need the support and understanding of GPs because there have been times when I have been desperate and suicidal and I am sure I am not alone.

Patient comment

Managing migraine is about more than making a diagnosis and providing a prescription. Drugs are necessary to treat migraine but the goal must be to help patients not to rely on medication alone. Tailoring management to meet individual needs can improve the outcome for the patient and reduce the number of consultations in the long term. The first step is to find out why the patient has sought help, then to make the diagnosis, followed by a discussion with the patient of possible management strategies.

The choice of appropriate medication, both for acute treatment and for prevention of attacks, is largely based on empirical evidence. Only a limited number of well-designed, controlled clinical trials have been undertaken, mostly with the 5-hydroxytryptamine 1D (5HT1D) agonist class of acute treatments. The suggestions below indicate common practice in the UK but are not intended to represent a professional standard in any given country.

Why has the patient come?

Although migraine is a common condition, most people have infrequent attacks that respond to over-the-counter treatments and they do not need to consult a doctor. Therefore, when patients do seek medical advice it is often for a specific reason that may be important to management.

Typical reasons include:
- increased frequency and/or severity of symptoms;
- failure of response to usual medication;
- change in symptoms;
- attacks are disrupting work/leisure;

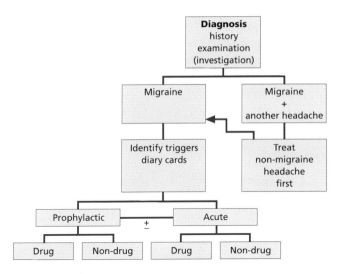

Fig. 8.1 Management plan.

- fear of serious illness;
- to discuss a new treatment they have read about.

By asking the questions: 'Why have you come to see me now?' and 'What worries you most about your headaches?' such management issues can be addressed early in the consultation.

Next is correct diagnosis of each headache, bearing in mind that the first four reasons for consulting listed above may be due to the development of a headache additional to migraine. Non-migraine headaches should be treated first because this in itself can reduce the frequency and severity of migraine (Fig. 8.1).

In the context of a correct diagnosis based on history and in the absence of neurological signs on examination, patients can be reassured that there is no evidence of a sinister cause for their headaches. It is worthwhile stating this as few patients directly voice their fears of an underlying brain tumour or stroke unless the doctor addresses it.

Discussing new remedies is a more difficult task. Patients arrive clutching newspaper cuttings about the latest miracle cure for migraine. Sometimes the treatments are valid and may be worth consideration. Alternative therapies are discussed later in this chapter.

Managing migraine

Management strategies can be divided into acute and prophylactic and further into drug and non-drug. Acute treatments are used to abort or reduce symptoms once an attack has started. If attacks are frequent prophylaxis may be considered, in addition to acute treatment. Identification and avoidance of predisposing and triggering factors may be sufficient to reduce attack frequency but occasionally a short course of drug prophylaxis is necessary. If prophylaxis is effective, attacks which break through are often less severe and more responsive to acute treatment. For drug use in pregnancy, see Chapter 10.

Acute treatment

Unlike a non-migraine headache, an attack of migraine is associated with gastrointestinal stasis and reduced rate of gastric emptying which can impair the absorption of drugs given orally.

It follows that acute management strategies should be instigated as early as possible in an attack. Early medication can abort an attack and minimize the total amount of drugs required, reducing potential side-effects.

Patients who recognize the early prodromal symptoms can sometimes abort an attack by avoiding known triggers, having an early night or even taking medication before they go to bed.

If prodromal symptoms are not present or not recognized, treatment should be taken at the onset of the migraine headache. Aura symptoms rarely respond to acute treatment although there is nothing to be lost by recommending the use of non-specific therapies such as analgesics or analgesic/antiemetic combinations at this time. However, it is uncertain if treatment taken at the onset of aura has any effect on the ensuing headache. Certainly, studies suggest that sumatriptan taken at the onset of aura has little effect on headache. This may not be the case with triptans which have central activity such as zolmitriptan but data are limited. Patients should be advised to carry at least a single dose of medication on them at all times so that there is no delay in treatment.

If treatment is delayed until the headache is established, drugs taken by mouth cannot be absorbed or drug absorption will be slower and reduced. Secondly, the analgesic activity of a drug is limited and if the level of pain exceeds the activity of the drug, then it will not be effective. It follows that treatment taken at the earliest recognized stage of an attack (before the onset of gastric stasis) will be the most effective.

Acute drug treatment

In a migraine attack give the right drug in the right dose at the right time and in the right form.

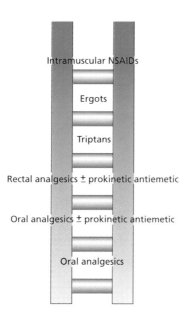

Fig. 8.2 Acute treatment ladder.

Before advising patients on medication it is useful to find out what they have taken in the past. If drugs have been taken too late in an attack or in an inadequate dose, it may be worth trying them again.

Since attacks vary in the same patient and in different patients, developing at different times of the day and building up to differing levels of severity, a treatment ladder is useful (Fig. 8.2). In practice this means that early, mild symptoms may be treated with simple analgesics but if the attack continues to develop treatments further up the ladder should be tried.

Patients are recommended to start at the lowest rung of the ladder that they think will be effective. If they recognize symptoms early and the attack builds up slowly, they should start with step one. If this proves ineffective after 1 or 2 h, they may try similar drugs as suppositories to circumvent gastric stasis (step 2). If this is also ineffective, they can move to either step 3 or step 4. If, after three attacks, they always need to shift up the ladder, treatment should be instigated from a higher step.

Different situations will also warrant different treatments. If an attack is fully developed with severe vomiting on waking, there is little point attempting take oral medication so either step 2 or a non-oral triptan would be more appropriate.

Limits to acute therapy: frequency of use

Overuse of acute medications can be associated with headaches that become refractory to acute and prophylactic treatments. Patients should be cautioned against using acute treatments regularly on more than 3 days a week. More frequent use is inappropriate for migraine and the true nature of the underlying headache(s) needs careful assessment.

Step 1A: oral analgesics (Table 8.1)

Simple over-the-counter oral analgesics such as aspirin, ibuprofen or paracetamol, are most frequently used. Efficacy can be improved by ensuring adequate doses are taken early in an attack before gastric stasis reduces absorption. Effervescent compounds are more rapidly absorbed. Some patients dissolve soluble analgesics in a sweet fizzy drink.

Many patients favour over-the-counter combinations such as Femigraine® (500 mg aspirin and 25 mg cyclizine), Migraleve® (pink: 500 mg paracetamol, 8 mg codeine and 6.25 mg buclizine; yellow: 500 mg paracetamol and 8 mg codeine) or Midrid® (325 mg paracetamol and 65 mg isometheptene mucate—a cerebral vasoconstrictor).

Non-steroidal anti-inflammatory drugs (NSAIDs) such as diclofenac, naproxen and tolfenamic acid may also be tried early in an attack. Their anti-inflammatory activity makes them particularly useful when muscle tenderness in the scalp or neck is a prominent symptom (Table 8.2).

Since there are no controlled clinical trials to support better efficacy, patients are best advised to use the cheapest drug which they find most effective.

Side-effects. These are generally few with episodic use. Paracetamol is particularly well tolerated in therapeutic doses but liver damage can follow overdose. Aspirin and NSAIDS may cause gastrointestinal

Table 8.1 Simple analgesics.

Analgesic	Dose (mg)	Max. daily (g)	Cost per dose (£)	Cost per max. daily dose (£)
Aspirin	600–900 every 4–6 h	4	Oral: 0.01 Rectal: 1.60–2.40	Oral: 0.05 Rectal: 9.50
Paracetamol	500–1000 every 4–6 h	4	Oral: 0.01 Rectal: 0.95–1.90	Oral: 0.04 Rectal: 7.60
Ibuprofen	400–800 every 4–6 h	2.4	Oral: 0.06–0.12	Oral: 0.36

Table 8.2 NSAIDs.

Analgesic	Dose (mg)	Max. daily (mg)	Cost per dose (£)	Cost per max. daily dose (£)
Diclofenac	Oral and rectal: 50 every 8–12 h	150	Oral: 0.06 Rectal: 0.21	Oral: 0.18 Rectal: 0.63
Naproxen	Oral and rectal: 250–500 every 12 h	1000	Oral: 0.06–0.11 Rectal: 0.16–0.32	Oral: 0.22 Rectal: 0.64
Tolfenamic acid	Oral: 200 repeat once after 2–3 h if necessary	400	Oral: 1.00	Oral: 2.00

discomfort, nausea, diarrhoea, and occasionally bleeding and ulceration. Gastric irritation may be minimized by taking these drugs with food and is less likely to occur with ibuprofen. They also cause generalized increased bleeding tendency and can be associated with hypersensitivity reactions including asthma, bronchospasm, dizziness, vertigo and tinnitus.

Cautions and contraindications. Aspirin and NSAIDS should be used with caution in the elderly and those with allergic disorders, renal, cardiac or hepatic disease. Doses should be kept as low as possible. Their use is contraindicated in patients with active peptic ulceration and concomitant use of histamine H2 receptor blocking drugs or misoprostol should be considered in patients at risk.

Relevant interactions. These include enhanced effect of anticoagulants, antagonism of the effects of antihypertensive drugs and increased risk of nephrotoxicity with thiazide diuretics.

Step 1B: oral analgesics plus oral domperidone or metoclopramide

Gastrointestinal symptoms are a common feature of migraine. Although over-the-counter antiemetic preparations are available and may be sufficient for some patients.

Domperidone and **metoclopramide** are the drugs of choice as, in addition to the antiemetic effect, they promote gastric emptying and normal peristalsis improving the absorption of analgesics during migraine (Fig. 8.3 & Table 8.3). They should be used even when patients are not nauseous in order to improve the efficacy of analgesics. In theory, domperidone or metoclopramide should be taken 10–15 min before analgesics; in practice, they can be taken concomitantly. Clinical trial

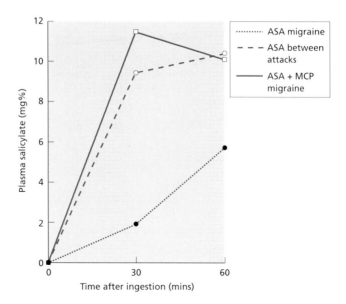

Fig. 8.3 Gastric stasis. Based on Volans GN. *Br J Clin Pharm* 1975; 2: 57–63.

data suggest that the combination of aspirin and metoclopramide is as effective as sumatriptan with fewer side-effects and obvious lower cost [1]. Combined analgesic/antiemetic preparations of Domperamol® (10 mg domperidone and 500 mg paracetamol), Migravess® (5 mg metoclopramide and 325 mg aspirin) and Paramax® (5 mg metoclopramide and 500 mg paracetamol) are available on prescription. It is important to note that although combinations have the advantage of convenience, they are more expensive than the individual drugs.

Side-effects. Metoclopramide may cause drowsiness. Its use can be associated with acute extrapyramidal reactions causing facial and skeletal muscle spasms and oculogyric crises. These symptoms usually occur shortly after taking a single dose and subside within 24 h. They can be aborted with a 1-mg intramuscular injection of benztropine.

Table 8.3 Pro-kinetic antiemetics.

Antiemetic	Dose (mg)	Max. daily (mg)	Cost per dose (£)	Cost per max. daily dose (£)
Domperidone	Oral: 20 every 4–8 h Rectal: 30–60 every 4–8 h	Oral: 80 Rectal: 120	Oral: 0.16 Rectal: 0.27–0.53	Oral: 0.64 Rectal: 1.06
Metoclopramide	10 every 8 h	30	Oral: 0.02	Oral: 0.06

Domperidone does not readily cross the blood–brain barrier so side-effects are rarely seen with episodic use.

Cautions and contraindications. Dystonic reactions following metoclopramide are more common in children and young women.

Relevant interactions. Concomitant use of antipsychotics can enhance extrapyramidal effects.

Step 2: change the route of administration

If gastrointestinal symptoms prohibit oral medication, drugs may be given rectally. Diclofenac or naproxen suppositories for pain, combined with domperidone if necessary, are recommended. It is often believed that patients in the UK find the idea of using suppositories distasteful. The author's experience is that, when asked, patients are prepared to use any route of delivery provided that it works. Explanation about using suppositories can help to dispel myths—and prevent the use of suppositories by the oral route! Although the apex foremost is the commonest method of insertion, patients are best advised to insert the base foremost. The latter method is associated with better retention, with no need to introduce a finger into the anal canal, and lower expulsion rate [2].

Addition to steps 1 and/or 2: short-acting benzodiazepine

Patients frequently state that they feel better when they sleep but pain prevents this. If necessary, sleep can be promoted by a short-acting seda-tive such as a single dose of 5–10 mg temazepam (note controlled drug requirements) or 0.5 mg lormetazepam. Provided hypnotics are given to patients with a clear diagnosis of migraine, who are carefully coun-selled about misuse, they will have little addictive potential.

Side-effects. Impaired judgement and increased reaction time affects the ability to drive or operate machinery. Some patients become confused or amnesic, others become aggressive.

Cautions and contraindications. Children and the elderly are more sensitive to side-effects. Avoid using in patients with respiratory disease and personality disorders.

Relevant interactions. The effects of alcohol are enhanced. Concomitant use of antidepressants or opioids enhances sedation. Hypnotics also enhance the hypotensive effect of antihypertensives.

Step 3: triptans (Table 8.4)

These drugs are selective 5HT1B/1D receptor agonist with selective vasoconstrictor properties; they are not analgesic. Although these drugs are specifically indicated for migraine, response does not confirm the diagnosis as they are effective for most vascular headaches.

Because of their different mode of action they can be used within an hour of lack of efficacy of earlier steps. Clinical trials suggest that triptans are effective whatever stage of the attack they are used; in practice they appear more effective if taken early. Recurrence of symptoms is a particular clinical problem for some patients, with migraine returning after initial response to treatment. This is typically the next day, but can occur later the same day. A few patients experience repeated episodes of recurrence over several consecutive days, sometimes extending the total duration of the attack to longer than an untreated attack. Recurrence appears to be an individual problem as patients who experience recurrence with one triptan are likely to have a similar problem with a different triptan. Recommendations for early treatment with triptans still apply as clinically symptoms are less likely to recur after initial response if attacks are aborted early.

Table 8.4 Triptans.

Triptan	Dose (mg)	Max./24 h (mg)	Cost per dose (£)	Cost per max. daily dose (£)
Naratriptan*				
Oral tablet	2.5	5	4.00	8.00
Sumatriptan*				
Oral tablet	50–100	300	4.70–8.00	24.00
Intranasal	20	40	8.00	16.00
Subcutaneous	6	12	19.57	39.14
Rizatriptan*				
Oral tablet	5–10	20	4.46	8.91
Oral lyophilisate (wafer)	10	20	4.46	8.91
Zolmitriptan†				
Oral tablet	2.5	15	4.00	24.00

*Repeat dose once in 24 h for recurrence only after initial response.
†Repeat dose 2 h after initial dose for lack of effect or recurrence.

Side-effects. Those which are typical to this class of drugs include dizziness, somnolence, asthenia and nausea. These are generally short-lived. 'Chest' symptoms, including tightness and pressure in the throat, neck and chest, are more common with sumatriptan than the other 'triptans'. The concern is that these symptoms are of cardiac origin. Although electrocardiographic studies rarely show changes suggestive of ischaemia, other than that associated with pre-existing disease, the cause of 'chest' symptoms remains unclear and caution is indicated [3].

'Chest' symptoms are of concern if:
- there is pain, rather than pressure, affecting the chest or arm;
- symptoms last longer than 60 min;
- symptoms begin to appear in later attacks, i.e. no symptoms were reported when the drug was used on the first few occasions;
- there is a history of cardiac risk factors (NB a contraindication to triptan use);
- there is a history of concurrent ergot use (NB a contraindication to triptan use).

8

Cautions and contraindications. These drugs should only be used when the diagnosis of migraine is established. Contraindications to this class of drugs are hypersensitivity, ischaemic heart disease, any condition associated with risk of stroke or coronary artery disease, prinzmetals angina/coronary vasospasm, peripheral vascular disease and uncontrolled hypertension. Use of vasoconstrictors is not recommended in elderly patients, even when apparently asymptomatic of vascular disease. Patients with potential unrecognized cardiovascular disease, for example postmenopausal women, males over age 40, patients with risk factors for coronary artery disease, diabetics and smokers, should not use triptans without prior evaluation (Table 8.5).

Relevant interactions. Concomitant use of other vasoconstrictor drugs such as ergotamine or other 5HT agonists should be avoided.

Sumatriptan (Imigran®)

This was the first triptan to be developed and is available in several forms: oral (50 mg, 100 mg), subcutaneous (6 mg) and intranasal (20 mg). In some countries it is also available in a 25-mg oral dose and as a suppository (25 mg). Relief from symptoms at 2 h can be up to 80% following a subcutaneous dose, and around 75% and 60% at 2 h following intranasal and oral doses, respectively. At 4 h, response rates are up to around 80% for the oral preparations. However, recurrence of headache

Table 8.5 Triptans: warnings.

	Renal impairment	Hepatic impairment	Driving/operating machinery	Children and adolescents	Over 65s	Pregnancy	Lactation
Naratriptan	C/I if severe i.e. creatinine clearance < 15 ml/min otherwise max. 2.5 mg/24 h	C/I if severe i.e. Child–Pugh grade C otherwise max. 2.5 mg/24 h	Caution but trials show no greater effect of Naramig than placebo	NR	NR	NR	NR
Sumatriptan	C/I if severe Caution if mild/moderate	C/I if severe 50-mg dose if mild/moderate	Caution	NR	NR	NR	NR
Rizatriptan	C/I if severe 5-mg dose if mild/moderate	C/I if severe 5-mg dose if mild/moderate	Caution— dizziness may occur	NR	NR	NR	Avoid breast feeding for 24 h after treatment
Zolmitriptan	No dose adjustment necessary	ID	Caution— somnolence may occur	NR	NR	NR	NR

C/I, contraindicated; NR, not recommended; ID, insufficient data.

has been reported to occur in about 40% of patients within 24 h of administration.

The subcutaneous dose has the advantage of rapid speed of onset but the disadvantage of more adverse events and earlier time to recurrence of symptoms. The nasal spray is convenient and easy to use and also acts faster than the tablet and suppository. For all forms of sumatriptan, a further dose should not be used if the first dose is not effective. However, if the migraine responds to the first dose but returns, a second dose can be used to treat the recurrent symptoms after a minimum interval of 2 h for the tablet or nasal spray and 1 h for the subcutaneous injection.

Side-effects. See general triptan data above.

Cautions and contraindications. See general triptan data above.

Specific interactions. In addition to the general 'triptan' interactions, sumatriptan should not be used concomitantly with monoamine oxidase inhibitors or within 2 weeks of discontinuation, selective 5HT re-uptake inhibitors or lithium. It should be avoided by patients with a sensitivity to sulphonamides. It should not be used until 24 h after ergotamine but ergotamine can be used 6 h after sumatriptan.

Naratriptan (Naramig®)

This is currently available only as an oral formulation (2.5 mg). In addition to its peripheral action on 5HT1 receptors, it is also thought to act centrally on the trigeminal nucleus caudalis in the brainstem. Compared with the other triptans, naratriptan has greater bioavailability and a longer half-life. It is better tolerated that sumatriptan with fewer reported adverse effects, including chest symptoms. Peak response is not seen until 4 h (up to 76%) and a repeat dose should not be used if there is no response to the first dose. However, a second dose may be taken at least 4 h after initial treatment if symptoms recur. The recurrence rate within 24 h is reported to be around 17–32%. Adverse events are fewer than with sumatriptan.

Adverse events. See general triptan data above.

Cautions and contraindications. See general triptan data above.

Specific interactions. In addition to the general 'triptan' interactions, naratriptan should not be used concomitantly with methysergide and should be avoided by patients with a sensitivity to sulphonamides. There is no interaction reported with monoamine oxidase inhibitors.

Rizatriptan (Maxalt®)

This also has central actions on the trigeminovascular system in addition to its peripheral properties. It is available as oral tablets (5 mg and 10 mg) and as an oral peppermint-flavoured lyophilisate (10 mg) which melts on the tongue. Rizatriptan has greater bioavailability compared with sumatriptan and a similar half-life. Absorption is delayed by about 1 h when the drug is taken with food. Response is reported half an hour after dosing. The 2-h response to 10 mg is around 67–77% compared with a placebo response of 23–40%. Recurrence within 24 h is between 30 and 47%.

Side-effects. See general triptan data above.

Cautions and contraindications. See general triptan data above.

Specific interactions. In addition to general triptan interaction, rizatriptan should not be used until 24 h after ergotamine but ergotamine can be used 6 h after rizatriptan. The 5-mg dose is recommended for patients taking propranolol. This interaction is not seen with atenolol, metoprolol, nadolol or timolol. It should not be used concomitantly with monoamine oxidase inhibitors or within 2 weeks of discontinuation. There is a theoretical interaction with selective serotonin re-uptake inhibitors (SSRIs) and CYP 2D6 substrates. Patients with phenylketonuria should be warned that the lyophilisate contains 2.10 mg phenylalanine.

Zolmitriptan (Zomig®)

This has central and peripheral actions. It is currently available as an oral preparation (2.5 mg). It has similar biovailability to rizatriptan but a slightly longer half-life. It has an active metabolite which contributes to the therapeutic effect. Response is reported within 1 h after dosing. The 2-h response to 2.5 mg is around 64% compared with a placebo response of 25%. Recurrence within 24 h is between 22 and 37%. An advantage of zolmitriptan is that a second 2.5-mg dose can be taken if symptoms persist 2 h after the initial dose. Subsequent attacks may then be treated with an initial 5-mg dose. If symptoms return more than 2 h after initial treatment, a repeat dose may be given.

Side-effects. See general triptan data above.

Cautions and contraindications. In addition to the general triptan contraindications, zolmitriptan should not be used patients with Wolff–Parkinson–White syndrome or dysrhythmias associated with other accessory pathways.

Specific interactions. In addition to general triptan interactions, a maximum intake of 7.5 mg in 24 h is recommended in patients taking monoamine oxidase inhibitors. It should not be used within 6 h of ergotamine. Other triptans may be used 12 h after zolmitriptan.

Triptans in practice (Table 8.6)

Clinical trial data should be interpreted with caution as although study designs were similar, differences in data recording and analysis make it difficult to compare data other than with results from comparative studies. Constraints of clinical trials are such that it is likely that the drugs are more effective in clinical practice than the trial data suggest. Further, patients often take triptans within a few hours of analgesics—an exclusion criterion for clinical trials. However, the results of clinical trials provide useful markers for efficacy and adverse events. Response in clinical trials is defined as improvement from severe of moderate to mild or no headache. A change from moderate to mild headache is of questionable significance. Further, placebo response can vary considerably. A more relevant parameter is response to no headache. With these limitations considered, there is the suggestion that 4 h efficacy is similar following oral doses of all available triptans. For 2 h oral data, rizatriptan and zolmitriptan appear to have faster onset to efficacy than sumatriptan, and naratriptan is slower. Adverse events are least with naratriptan and most with sumatriptan. Recurrence is least with naratriptan.

If gastrointestinal disturbance or other symptoms preclude oral therapy, or if a patient requires rapid onset to efficacy, intranasal and subcutaneous sumatriptan are first and second line, respectively.

Table 8.6 Triptans.

Oral drugs	Speed of onset	Recurrence in 24 h	Side-effects
Naratriptan 2.5 mg	+	+	+
Sumatriptan 100 mg	++	+++	+++
Rizatriptan 10 mg	++++	+++	++
Zolmitriptan 2.5 mg	+++	++	++

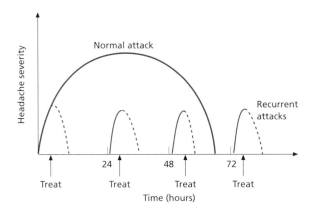

Fig. 8.4 Recurrence of migraine.

Rizatriptan wafers are convenient to use when a drink is not available or when nausea or vomiting is a problem. However, absorption is slower than the tablets, delaying onset to efficacy.

Postmarketing studies will provide more robust comparative data and establish the place of rizatriptan. Data from comparative studies with the promising newer triptans, including almotriptan, eletriptan, and frovatriptan, will help establish their future role in clinical practice.

Treatment of recurrence after initial efficacy within same attack
(Fig. 8.4)

A second dose of the same triptan is usually effective but may not be the most appropriate treatment, particularly for long-duration attacks where recurrence may occur repeatedly over several days. **Diclofenac** oral or suppository may be tried instead, perhaps pre-emptively where recurrence is usual and expected. If it is a continuing problem, drugs with a long half-life, such as ergotamine or dihydroergotamine, may be appropriate.

Combining triptans or ergotamine with analgesics and antiemetics

There is no evidence of adverse interaction between triptans and the drugs used in earlier steps. This means that triptans can be taken concomitantly with antiemetics, although there are no data to show whether or not this enhances therapeutic response. Similarly, analgesics may also be used concomitantly. Combining drugs has the potential advantage of treating the migraine by three different mechanisms but the disadvantage of increasing the likelihood of side-effects.

Table 8.7 Ergotamine.

Route	Dose	Max. doses/week*	Cost per dose (£)
Oral	1–2 mg	2	0.04‡; 0.29–0.58†
Rectal	1–2 mg (half to one suppository)	2	0.08–0.16§
Inhalation	1–3 × 0.36-mg metered doses	6 metered doses	0.04**

*Author's recommendation.
†Migril (Glaxo Wellcome) = ergotamine tartrate 2 mg, cyclizine hydrochloride 50 mg, caffeine 100 mg.
‡Cafergot (Sandoz) = ergotamine tartrate 1 mg, caffeine 100 mg.
§Cafergot (Sandoz) = ergotamine tartrate 2 mg, caffeine 100 mg.
**Medihaler-ergotamine (3M) = ergotamine tartrate 0.36 mg per dose.

8

Step 4: ergotamine and dihydroergotamine (Tables 8.7 & 8.8)

Ergotamine

This has been prescribed for migraine since the 1920s. It has non-selective 5HT and α-adrenergic activity resulting in non-selective vasoconstrictor effects. Carefully used, it can be a very effective treatment and may be tried if recurrence with triptan use is a particular problem as the biological half-life is considerably longer than that of the triptans. Data on comparative studies with sumatriptan have limited clinical relevance as oral ergotamine was used. Oral ergotamine has very poor and variable bioavailability (< 1%) and is not recommended. Per rectum or inhalations are the preferred routes of delivery with a bioavailability of 1–3%. A persistent vasoconstrictor effect, for at least 24 h, follows a single therapeutic dose of ergotamine. Ideally, treatment should not be repeated after the initial dose for a further 4 days, with a maximum of two doses per week.

Table 8.8 Dihydroergotamine.

Route	Dose	Max. dose/week*	Cost per dose (£)
Intranasal	1–2 × 2-mg metered doses	4 metered doses	N/A

*Author's recommendation.
N/A, not available at time of writing.

Side-effects. These include nausea, vomiting, cold peripheries, muscle aches and general malaise. It has a narrow therapeutic window so the dose should be titrated against symptoms, starting with a low dose. Patients should also be counselled about misuse which can result in daily headache or even ergotism with thrombosis and gangrene. Ergotamine should not be used in children or the elderly.

Cautions and contraindications. These are similar to the triptans but greater caution is recommended because of toxicity with high doses and the potential of ergotism with continued misuse. Ergotamine is not an option if triptans are contraindicated.

Relevant interactions. Ergotamine should not be used if the attack has already been treated with a triptan, and vice versa, but may be used in future attacks. Concomitant use of β-blockers or erythromycin should be avoided as their use can potentiate ergotism.

Dihydroergotamine

This is reported to be as effective as ergotamine with a low incidence of recurrence (< 20%), probably due to its long half-life of 10 h. Its advantage over ergotamine is that is has fewer adverse effects. It is given as a subcutaneous or intramuscular injection, or by inhalation. In the UK it is only available as a nasal spray. One metered dose should be used in each nostril (i.e. total of two doses) at the onset of an attack. An additional one to two doses can be repeated after a minimum of 15 min for lack of response. Treatment may be repeated after an interval of 8 h to a maximum of eight metered doses in 24 h. Although the data sheet allows a maximum weekly dose of 24 metered doses, the author recommends that treatment should be restricted to 2 days per week, with a maximum of eight metered doses per week.

Side-effects. Side-effects specific to the intranasal route include bad taste and local nasal symptoms such as rhinitis, stuffy nose and flushing. Other reactions include nausea and vomiting, numbness and tingling in fingers and toes, and chest tightness.

Cautions and contraindications. Contraindications are similar to the triptans and ergotamine. It should not be used in patients with severe hepatic impairment. Heavy smokers should not use dihydroergotamine because of the increased risk of vasoconstriction.

Relevant interactions. Concomitant use of macrolide antibiotics such as erythromycin should be avoided since they may increase the plasma level of dihydroergotamine. Concomitant use of ergotamine and triptans is also contraindicated. β-blockers should be avoided in patients susceptible to vasoconstriction.

Step 5: intramuscular diclofenac

Self-injected intramuscular 75 mg diclofenac may be worth trying but is not common practice. It is difficult as the intramuscular volume is 3 ml and may require two sites. There is also the risk of sterile abscesses.

Drugs for the doctor's bag: emergency treatment

Since most patients with migraine visit their doctor between attacks, when they are well, it is not uncommon for some patients to request a home visit in order to show the doctor how ill they really are during an attack. Home visits for migraine need to be carefully handled. The diagnosis needs to be confirmed, particularly if symptoms are atypical or different from the patients usual attacks. It is important to ensure that patients do not become dependent on such management for future attacks as they may label themselves as unresponsive to more simple management strategies and be conditioned to expect a home visit for future attacks. Suppositories can be given if not already used (see step 2 above). Intramuscular **diclofenac** 75 mg and/or intramuscular **chlorpromazine** 25–50 mg (potent antiemetic and sedative) may be tried. Intramuscular or even intravenous **metoclopramide** 10 mg is another option if the patient has tolerated oral metoclopramide in the past, although extrapyramidal effects are more common with this route. Intravenous **aspirin** is used in some countries but is not available in the UK. Although very effective opiate drugs such as pethidine are best avoided (see below). Early follow-up is recommended and patients should be asked to make an appointment to review their migraine when they have recovered.

'Long-duration' migraine

Attacks lasting more than 3 days are rarely solely due to migraine. One cause to consider is repeated recurrence from triptans which should be suspected if symptoms are responding to a dose of a triptan but require repeated doses on consecutive days. Since typical migraine is usually followed by a refractory period of 2 or 3 days before a new attack can develop, such attacks are recurrence of the same migraine which has only temporarily responded to treatment. Recurrence can occur for up to 5 or 6 days. Another cause is that the migraine is superseded by a tension-type headache, typically muscle contraction. The history will elicit muscle pain in the neck and shoulder and improvement of nausea and vomiting. In either case, try **diclofenac** by any route. If such attacks are a continuing problems and response to any therapy is poor, review the diagnosis and consider medication misuse.

Slowly developing migraine

Some patients develop attacks slowly and initially are uncertain if a headache is migrainous or not. **Steps one or two** are recommended at this stage. As there is some evidence that delayed use of **triptans** does not significantly impair efficacy, triptans should not be used until it is certain that the headache is migrainous.

Drugs to avoid in acute intervention

Opiates or opiate derivatives (including codeine, dihydrocodeine and pethidine) increase nausea, promote systemic shut-down and have addictive potential. Patients may feel that their migraine is 'too severe' to respond to other drugs for future attacks, increasing the call-out rate and making long-term management difficult.

Barbiturates are popular for migraine in some countries although are rarely used in the UK. They have limited efficacy and have addictive potential.

When acute treatments fail

Therapeutic failure is often due to an insufficient dose of the right drug, delayed treatment, the right drug given by the wrong route or even use of the wrong drug. If nothing works after these factors have been considered, review the diagnosis.

Acute non-drug treatment

Simple strategies can be effective in their own right as well as enhancing the efficacy of acute drug treatments.
- Recommend to patients that they always carry with them at least one dose of medication so that treatment is not delayed.
- Treatment is best taken with a drink or light carbohydrate snack.

8

- Sleep can aid recovery so patients should be advised to sit or rest somewhere quiet, even if only for a short time.
- Ice- or heat-pads on the site of pain may provide some relief.
- Acupressure, massage and biofeedback can be tried.

Prophylaxis

The aim of prophylaxis is to reduce the frequency and severity of attacks. Long-term strategies include lifestyle changes, and removing or avoiding predisposing and precipitating factors. Migraine is a long-standing condition in most patients seeking medical advice, therefore a change in the pattern is unlikely to take place overnight. In the short term, courses of prophylactic medication may be indicated for frequent attacks when acute therapy alone fails to provide adequate symptom control.

Predisposing factors

There are several factors that predispose to increased frequency of migraine which can be picked up from the history and examination. Each of these requires specific intervention which may be sufficient to enable the patient to manage the migraine without further action:

- anxiety and depression;
- head or neck trauma;
- illness;
- drugs;
- medication misuse;
- side-effect of drugs taken for other conditions.

Precipitating factors

Many patients state that they have given up eating cheese and chocolate in an effort to prevent migraine. In practice, such foods are more likely to induce migraine through fear of eating them than by any recognized biochemical process. Few patients are aware of more important migraine triggers such as missed meals or sleeping in which are discussed in more detail in Chapter 6.

Identifying relevant trigger factors can help reduce the frequency of migraine attacks by up to 50%—similar to the efficacy of the popular prophylactic drug pizotifen. Patients must be motivated since the process can be time consuming and it may be several months before possible causes and effects are noticed; it is not a suitable method for patients

May	Day	Headache	Time started	How long it lasted	Did you feel sick	Were you sick	What tablets did you take	What time taken	What triggered the attack
1	Tue								
2	Wed								
3	Thu								
4	Fri								
5	Sat								
6	Sun								
7	Mon								
8	Tue	Severe	4 pm	All night	Yes	Yes	Domperidone (1) Aspirin (3)	} 4 & 10 pm	Missed lunch Went shopping
9	Wed	Moderate	"	All night	Yes	No	"	8 am	
10	Thu								
11	Fri								
12	Sat								
13	Sun								
14	Mon								

Fig. 8.5 'Attack' diaries can aid diagnosis and help identify triggers.

wanting 'instant' prophylaxis. However, it does provide patients with a unique insight into their own attacks which can lead to more effective long-term control. Diary cards are the key to success so it is essential that patients understand how to complete them accurately, with as much information as possible.

The 'attack' diary (Fig. 8.5)

Attack diaries, in addition to their value in diagnosis, can also help identify triggers. The patient should be asked to record all different headaches on the diary card, in addition to all medication taken, for whatever reason. Women should keep a record of their menstrual periods, premenstrual symptoms and hormonal treatments such as oral contraception or hormone replacement therapy.

For each headache the following should be recorded, as a minimum:
• date;
• day of the week;
• time attack started;
• associated symptoms;
• duration of symptoms;
• treatment used, including dose and time taken.

The diary card should be reviewed after 3 months. A record of migraine will show attacks occurring episodically with days in between when the patient is headache free. If the patient has daily headaches, the diary may show symptoms of migraine superimposed on the daily headache.

The diary can highlight timing of attacks. If attacks occur early in the morning, late morning or late afternoon, it is useful to ask about the time of meals, as such attacks are often related to missed meals. Eating a snack at bedtime, mid-morning or mid-afternoon may be the only treatment that is necessary to prevent attacks. A link with sleeping in at weekends, or with regular commitments such as a long car journey once a week, or visit to the gym, may also be noted.

The diary card will also show if the correct treatment is being taken at the right time, in the right form and in the right dose. If acute treatment is being taken frequently, on more than 2–3 days each week, consider medication misuse.

The trigger diary (Table 8.9)

8

If patients have frequent attacks of migraine, more than once a month, they may find keeping a trigger diary useful, in addition to the attack diary.

Triggers appear to be cumulative, reaching a 'threshold' above which attacks are initiated. Therefore, rather than **'What** triggers an attack?', a more useful question is **'How many** triggers initiate an attack?'.

Patients can be given a list of typical triggers and asked to record all potential triggers present each day, even when they do not have a migraine.

Treat triggers: 'moderation in all things'

The daily trigger diary and the attack diary should be reviewed after at least five attacks. Compare the information in each, looking for a build-up of triggers coinciding with the attacks.

Table 8.9 Attack and trigger diaries.

Identify prodromal symptoms
Identify optimum time for treatment
Identify adequate medication
Identify triggers
Relationship to meals/sleep/activities
Identify pattern
'Weekend' migraine/'menstrual' migraine/
'pill-free' interval/progestogens

Not every trigger applies to every patient and different triggers may be responsible for different attacks in the same patient. It is unnecessary and impractical to attempt to avoid all migraine triggers but give general advice to eat regularly, maintain a regular sleep pattern, avoid getting overtired, and take regular exercise. To identify specific triggers, ask patients to study the list and divide them into two groups—those which they can do something about (e.g. missing meals, sleeping in) and those which are out of their control (e.g. menstrual cycle, travelling). They should first try to deal with the triggers that they have some influence over, cutting out suspect triggers one at a time. Triggers can be balanced—if patients are having a particularly stressful time, they should take extra care to eat regularly and avoid excessive intake of stimulants such as tea, coffee and alcohol.

Drug prevention (Table 8.10)

Prophylactic drugs are not curative but can help the patient regain control during periods of frequent and severe migraine attacks. Most prophylactics only reduce the frequency of migraine by around 50% at best, compared with placebo [4]. One reason for this may be poor compliance with migraine prophylaxis, particularly if more than once- or twice-daily doses are used [5]. The majority are not specific to migraine and are usually effective in doses lower than required for their more usual indications. Prophylactic drugs should not be used long-term as migraine is a remitting condition. Acute treatment is still necessary for breakthrough attacks.

Table 8.10 Prophylactic drugs.

Drug	Starting dose (mg)	Max. daily (mg)	Cost per 28 days: start dose (£)	Cost per 28 days: max. dose (£)
β-blocker, e.g. propranolol	10 twice daily	240 in three divided doses (long-acting once daily)	0.14	0.59 12.07
Amitriptyline*	10 nocte	75 nocte	0.18	0.38
Pizotifen	0.5 nocte	3 nocte	2.18	15.56
Sodium valproate*	200 twice daily	1000 in divided doses	3.58	8.82
Mesthysergide	1 nocte	2 three times daily	2.50	15.02

*Not licensed for migraine in the UK.

94

How to prescribe prophylaxis

- Do not assume that patients want to take prophylaxis. Consider their views, perhaps by asking 'How would you feel about taking a tablet every day to help prevent your migraine?'. Some may wish to try non-drug methods first.
- Explain possible early side-effects, indicating when improvement might be expected.
- Treatments should be restricted to episodes of exacerbation of attacks and can usually be withdrawn gradually after 4–6 months.
- Use once- or twice-daily doses where possible, to aid compliance.
- The lowest possible initial dose is recommended which should be gradually increased at 2–4-week intervals until symptoms are controlled or side-effects limit use.
- The highest dose tolerated should be continued for 2 months before the drug is deemed ineffective although, in practice, few patients will persevere for so long.
- If attacks fail to respond, try an alternative prophylactic. Question the diagnosis for repeated lack of response to different drugs.

8

Which prophylactic?

There is no single drug which is best for migraine prophylaxis. Each patient has different needs. The choice of drug is based on an empirical balance of risk vs. benefit for each patient (Tables 8.11 & 8.12). Combinations are not recommended as there is little evidence of enhanced

Table 8.11 Prophylaxis.

β-blockers
Hypertensive/stress/muscle tension
  10–40 mg bd

Amitriptyline
Poor sleep/depression
Additional headaches
  10–50 mg 2 h before bedtime

Pizotifen
Children/poor appetite
  0.5–1.5 mg 2 h before bedtime

Sodium valproate
Additional headaches
  200–500 mg bd

Table 8.12 Prophylactic drugs.

Drug	Side-effects	Contraindications
β-blocker, e.g. propranolol	Bradycardia, heart failure, bronchospasm	Heart failure, asthma
Amitriptyline*	Dry mouth, sedation, dizziness, nausea	Recent myocardial infarction, heart block, mania
Pizotifen	Weight gain, drowsiness	Urinary retentions, closed angled glaucoma
Sodium valproate*	Weight gain, hair loss, gastrointestinal disturbance, bruising	Hepatic disease, thrombocytopenia
Methysergide	Retroperitoneal and other abnormal fibrotic reactions, arterial spasm, postural hypotension	Renal, hepatic, pulmonary and cardiovascular disease, collagen disorders

*Not licensed for migraine in the UK.

efficacy and greater likelihood of side-effects. In general, the most commonly used first-line agents are β-adrenergic blockers.

First-line prophylactic agents

β-adrenergic blockers without partial agonism (Table 8.13)

Atenolol, metoprolol, nadolol, propranolol and timolol have all shown efficacy in clinical trials although atenolol is not licensed for migraine

Table 8.13 β-blockers.

	Start dose (mg)	Max. daily (mg)	Cost per 28 days: start dose (£)	Cost per 28 days: max. dose (£)
β-blocker,	25 once daily	200	2.46	2.50
Metroprolol	50 twice daily 100 long-acting once daily	200	1.96 2.28	3.78 4.56
Nadolol	40 once daily	160	3.46	10.90
Metroprolol	10 twice daily	240 (long-acting once daily)	0.14	0.59 12.07
Timolol	10 once daily	20	2.39	4.79

*Not licensed for migraine in the UK.

in the UK. There is no evidence that any of these drugs is more effective than the other. Therefore the choice depends on dosing regimens, side-effects, efficacy and cost. Atenolol and nadolol, with long half-lives can be administered once daily. The mechanism of action in migraine is obscure.

Failure to respond to one β-blocker does not predict failure to respond to another so several different β-blockers may be tried consecutively.

Indications. These drugs are particularly useful if there is associated hypertension or anxiety.

Dose. The lowest effective dose, preferably with a maximum twice-daily dosing regimen.

Side-effects. These include insomnia despite fatigue, and vivid dreams and cold extremities are fairly common, particularly in higher doses.

Contraindications. These include asthma, brittle diabetes, chronic obstructive airways disease, congestive cardiac failure, second or third atrioventricular block, peripheral vascular disease and Raynaud's disease.

Interactions. These include concomitant use of ergotamine. Use of the combined oral contraceptive pill may antagonize a required hypotensive effect.

Amitriptyline

Amitriptyline inhibits serotonin re-uptake at central synapses resulting in antidepressant properties. The antimigraine effect, however, appears to be unrelated to its antidepressant action.

Indications. It is particularly useful if there is associated depression, sleep disturbance and tension-type headache.

Dose. Initially 10 mg taken 2 h before bedtime which may be increased, as necessary by 10 mg every 2 weeks to a maximum of 150 mg in divided doses. It is rarely necessary to use doses higher than 75 mg *nocte* unless the patient is depressed.

Side-effects. Include sedation, dry mouth, dizziness, weight changes, constipation, urinary retention, blurred vision. Many of these effects,

8

particularly sedation, improve after the first 2 weeks of treatment. Patients should be warned that there may be no benefit noted for the first few weeks.

Contraindications. These include acute myocardial infarction, heart block, closed-angle glaucoma.

Interactions. These include monoamine oxidase inhibitors (concomitantly or within 14 days of use), other antidepressives, carbamazepine, phenytoin, alcohol. Use of the combined oral contraceptive pill may antagonize a required antidepressant effect and may increase side-effects.

Pizotifen

Pizotifen is an antihistamine and serotonin antagonist structurally related to the tricyclic antidepressants.

Indications. It is particularly useful if poor sleep or poor appetite are also a problem.

Dose. Initially 0.5 mg 2 h before bedtime increasing to 1.5–3 mg *nocte*. It is rarely necessary to give additional daytime doses.

Side-effects. These include sedation and weight gain. The latter is a particular issue for many women.

Contraindications. These include caution in patients with glaucoma or urinary retention. Avoid using in obese patients.

Interactions. Pizotifen antagonizes the hypotensive effect of adrenergic neurone blockers.

Sodium valproate

This is one of the few prophylactic agents which has undergone controlled clinical trials. It is speculated that its mode of action in migraine may be due to its action on γ-aminobutyric acid (GABA) receptors, or by its effect on reducing levels of the excitatory amino acid glutamate in the central nervous system.

Indications. Particularly useful if the patient has additional tension-type headache.

98

Dose. Initially 200 mg twice daily increasing to a daily dose of 1000 mg in divided doses. Serum levels should be between 50 and 120 mg/l but it is rarely necessary to measure these in clinical practice unless compliance or lack of effect needs to be checked.

Side-effects. These include weight gain, hair loss, gastrointestinal disturbance, bruising.

Contraindications. These include hepatic disease and thrombocytopenia. It may be necessary to check liver function and clotting before prescribing valproate. Because of the high incidence of fetal malformations, women should be using effective contraception.

Interactions. These include aspirin (enhances effect of valproate by displacing it from its binding sites—this can lead to toxicity) and cimetidine (increases plasma valproate). Antidepressants antagonize the anticonvulsant effect which is important if the patient is also taking valproate for epilepsy.

8

Second-line prophylactic drugs

Methysergide

This derivative of ergot has serotonin receptor antagonist activity.

Indications. Methysergide is specific for migraine prophylaxis and its use should be restricted to severe cases which have failed to respond to alternative therapies. Although it is very effective, potential side-effects affect up to 40% of users. Rarely, retroperitoneal, heart valve and pleural fibrosis are associated with use. Although there is no means of routinely monitoring for the development of fibrosis, it is not known to occur if a 1-month break from treatment is taken in every 6 months of use. These concerns mean that its use is usually only recommended on the advice of a specialist.

Dose. Initially 1 mg/day increasing by 1 mg every 3 days until response is achieved or to maximum 2 mg three times daily. To minimize the risk of fibrosis, the patient should be instructed to stop therapy for at least 1 month after each 6 months of use, gradually reducing the dose during the previous 2–3 weeks.

Side-effects. These include nausea, dyspepsia, leg cramps, dizziness, sedation.

Contraindications. These include peripheral vascular disease, severe hypertension, cardiac disease, impaired hepatic or renal function.

Interactions. These include ergot alkaloids and other vasoconstrictor drugs.

Other drugs used for prophylaxis

Calcium channel antagonists

Indications. Although widely used in some countries, they are of doubtful value. Only flunarizine has shown some efficacy and is not available in the UK. Verapamil is occasionally used by some specialists but the scientific proof for efficacy is limited.

Dose. Flunarizine 5–10 mg once daily (usually *mane*); 240–480 mg daily verapamil in divided doses or slow-release preparation.

Side-effects. These include sedation, dizziness, nausea and vomiting. Flunarizine is associated with depression and extrapyramidal symptoms.

Contraindications. These include personal or close family history of depression. Verapamil should not be used if there is second- or third-degree atrioventricular block, severe bradycardia or severe hypotension.

Interactions. Concomitant use of β-blockers is contraindicated.

Clonidine

Indications. Originally a centrally acting α-adrenoceptor agonist indicated for hypertension, clonidine has shown limited efficacy for migraine prophylaxis. It may have a place in the management of menopausal women with migraine and hot flushes who do not wish to take hormone replacement therapy.

Dose. Twenty-five to fifty micrograms three times daily.

Side-effects. These include sedation, dry mouth, dizziness, depression.

Contraindications. These include history of severe depression.

Interactions. These include antihypertensives.

Cyproheptadine

This is an antihistamine with serotonin-antagonist and calcium-channel-blocking properties.

Indications. May be useful when additional sedation is of benefit.

Dose. A 4-mg night-time dose is usually sufficient.

Side-effects. These include dry mouth, blurred vision, sedation and weight gain. Hypersensitivity reactions have been reported.

Contraindications. These include caution if used in epilepsy, urinary retention, glaucoma and hepatic disease.

Interactions. These include an enhanced sedative effect with alcohol and antidepressants. Concomitant use of other antihistamines should be avoided.

Non-steroidal anti-inflammatory drugs

Indications. NSAIDs can be useful if muscle contraction is present particularly if it is a possible triggering factor.

Dose. Diclofenac 75 mg twice daily; ibuprofen 400–600 mg three times daily; mefenamic acid 250–500 mg three times daily; naproxen 500 mg twice daily. Usually a 1–2-month course is sufficient to break the cycle of attacks. Treatment should be discontinued if no efficacy is evident after 2 weeks on the maximum dose.

Side-effects. These include dyspepsia, diarrhoea, peptic ulceration, dizziness, blood dyscrasias, hypersensitivity reactions.

Contraindications. These include aspirin/NSAID-induced asthma, active peptic ulcer, bleeding disorders. Aspirin is contraindicated in the UK for children under age 12 because of the risk of Reye's syndrome.

Interactions. These include anticoagulants, lithium, β-blockers, angiotensin-converting enzyme (ACE) inhibitors, methotrexate, frusemide, probenecid, quinolones, sulphonylureas, lithium, hydantoins.

Selective serotonin re-uptake inhibitors (SSRIs)

Indications. Clinical trials evidence of efficacy of fluoxetine in migraine is inconclusive but it may have a place if there is associated depression and the sedative effects of amitriptyline are unwanted or if there are symptoms of the premenstrual syndrome. SSRIs are not licensed for the treatment of migraine in the UK.

Dose. Fluoxetine 20 mg alternate days increasing to 40 mg daily.

Side-effects. These include nausea, vomiting, diarrhoea, weight gain, insomnia, anxiety and allergic reactions.

Contraindications. These include severe renal failure and unstable epilepsy.

Interactions. These include sumatriptan, monoamine oxidase inhibitors, tricyclic antidepressants, carbamazepine, phenytoin.

What if it fails?

Prophylactic drugs should not be discontinued until an adequate dose has been tried for an adequate duration. This is usually a minimum of 2 weeks at the highest dose that does not produce unacceptable side-effects. An alternative prophylactic can be tried in the same way. One important factor to review is compliance as a surprising number of patients do not even get the prescription filled or stop after a few days of treatment because of side-effects or lack of response. The wrong diagnosis is another possibility. Failure to respond to any prophylactic therapy is often associated with misuse of acute treatments.

Using drugs that are not licensed for migraine

In the UK a Product Licence is necessary before a medicine can be marketed for human use [6]. This is a constraint for the Pharmaceutical Industry but does not restrict doctors from using drugs for unlicensed indications. This is relevant to migraine as many of the drugs recommended are not licensed for migraine, despite their common usage. This has some practical implications as it increases the doctor's professional responsibility. In the event of a mishap a patient may seek compensation either by proving negligence liability or strict liability. The following points should be considered before a drug is prescribed outside its licensed indications.

• Ensure that the medication is being used in a way that would be endorsed by a responsible body of professional opinion.
• Write in the notes that the medicine is unlicensed for use.
• Inform the patient of the medicine's license status.
• Inform the patient of benefits and potential side-effects of the medicine, where possible in sufficient detail to allow the patient to give informed consent. Document in the notes that this has been done. A handout can be useful in these circumstances.

Alternative therapies

8

Nearly 70% of migraine sufferers have tried 'alternative' medical treatments at some time. Many help to reduce the effects of triggers, especially neck and back problems. Most of the following treatments are not available on the NHS. Homeopathy, osteopathy and physiotherapy have limited availability. An increasing number of GPs practice acupuncture. The cost of private treatment can vary considerably. Complementary medicine can be used as an adjunct, rather than as an alternative, to conventional treatment. Results of studies should be considered with caution as the nature of the treatment makes placebo-controlled studies difficult. This is particularly important as the close relationship between the patient and the practitioner, and the 'holistic' approach adopted, is likely to result in a high placebo response.

Acupuncture

Several published studies have shown acupuncture to be an effective migraine prophylactic. The results of one study suggest that acupuncture may be equipotent to the β-blocker metoprolol in reducing the frequency and duration, but not the severity, of attacks [7].

Alexander technique

This technique was introduced by F.M. Alexander (1869–1955) who felt that bad posture could cause pain and illness. The emphasis is on unlearning bad habits of movement and to correct the relationship between the head and neck to the rest of the body. Such treatment may be of specific help to headache sufferers with stiff and tender neck muscles.

Biofeedback

Biofeedback is particularly popular in the United States. There are several publications suggesting its efficacy in migraine. In one study, 74% of 63 migraine sufferers improved, as assessed by a decrease in headache severity as well as in the type and dose of analgesics used.

A meta-analysis of trials using propranolol and relaxation/biofeedback training for the treatment of migraine found that both treatments produced similar results [8].

Stress management, counselling and psychotherapy

Everyone has problems in life but not everyone is able to deal with them. Psychotherapy can help identify these stresses and help the patient find ways of coming to terms with them. Since stress and anxiety can trigger migraine attacks, some patients have found this treatment beneficial. Hypnosis techniques have also shown some efficacy.

Homeopathy

The principle of homeopathy is to treat like with like. Patients are prescribed minute amounts of substances that can imitate the symptoms of the illness. The substances recommended depend on the precise symptoms of each individual so two people with similar problems may be given different treatments. Homeopathic treatments should only be taken on the advice of a qualified practitioner. There are several NHS homeopathic hospitals in the UK. Although homeopathy may be effective for some conditions, controlled clinical trials of homeopathy in migraine show limited efficacy [9].

Massage

As a means of reducing tension in the muscles and providing an indulgent method of relaxation, massage can be very helpful. If performed regularly, massage can help minimize the headaches resulting from stress. Some find massage combined with aromatic oils (aromatherapy) particularly beneficial as oils can be used to ease specific problems including poor sleep or sinus pain.

Orthodontic treatment

Migraine and non-migraine headaches are not infrequently associated with tenderness over the temples and temporomandibular joints. It is worth asking the opinion of a dentist or orthodontist particularly if the jaw locks out or if the patient grinds their teeth at night and wakes with migraine.

Osteopathy and chiropractic

Osteopaths and chiropractors can help treat local pain in the head and neck, if this is a suspected trigger for attacks. Chiropractors believe many diseases are the result of disturbed spinal function and focus more specifically on the axial skeleton.

Physiotherapy

Chartered physiotherapists can also help relieve local muscle pains. Some physiotherapists are qualified in acupuncture, electrotherapy, and manual therapy, in addition to giving lifestyle training and advice.

Phytotherapy

Patients who dislike taking drugs may be happy to try herbal preparations. To many people, herbal treatment implies 'safe treatment', which is not necessarily true. Feverfew (*Tanacetum parthenium*) is the commonest herbal remedy for migraine and the results of prospective clinical trials in previous users of feverfew support its prophylactic efficacy.

The active ingredient was thought to be parthenolide which inhibits prostaglandin synthesis and platelet aggregation by a mechanism that is independent of cyclo-oxygenase. However, clinical trials using parthenolide extracted from feverfew have not shown promising results. The effective agent remains obscure. Feverfew can be taken in any form (dried or fresh leaves, tablet or liquid form) but may take up to 6 weeks before taking effect. One recommended dose is two to three fresh leaves or 50–100 mg dried feverfew daily. It has a bitter taste best disguised in a sandwich or salad.

Side-effects are few and rarely serious but the patient should be warned of the possibility of mouth ulcers, sore tongue, abdominal pain or indigestion. Feverfew should not be taken in pregnancy as it can stimulate endometrial muscle. Long-term effects are unknown but feverfew does contain sesquiterpene lactones which are highly reactive and possess cytotoxic activity *in vitro*.

The cost of treating migraine

Healthcare budgets are becoming increasingly stretched and the new acute treatments are not cheap. However, the recommendations above make it clear that in some cases migraine may be managed with cheaper therapies, reserving the triptans for specific occasions. Attitudes to self-medication are changing and more patients are aware that prescription drugs are not always necessary. This can reduce the cost of treatment for both doctor and patient. So do not be afraid to recommend over-the-counter therapies, if appropriate, but provide specific instructions on how to optimize efficacy.

Beware misuse: patients regularly using acute headache treatments on more than 2 days a week are not just breaking your budget, they are receiving inappropriate treatment. Reassess the diagnosis, and consider the need for prophylaxis. Although acute treatments for breakthrough attacks will still be needed, effective prophylaxis will reduce the frequency of use and symptoms may become more responsive to cheaper drugs. But when considering costs, it is necessary to include the benefits of effective treatment for the patient. For many people it has made the difference between losing 2 or 3 days from work and consequent fear of losing their job, and being able to continue to function. It can also improve the quality of life between attacks, by removing the fear of the next migraine.

Case study

Derek, aged 36, had attacks of common migraine two to three times a month, following a neck injury. He followed the doctor's advice and, with acupuncture to prevent attacks, had managed to reduce the frequency of migraine to one attack every 6–8 weeks. However, although the analgesic/antiemetic combination his doctor had recommended was usually effective, he would occasionally lose a day from work. This is particularly the case when he wakes with migraine, as the symptoms are much more severe than attacks which gradually develop during the day. The doctor suggests that Derek should start with his usual treatment for most attacks, but if this is not effective within an hour or if the attack is severe, he can try another treatment. Derek is not keen to use suppositories so the doctor suggests a triptan. Derek only has mild nausea and so the doctor prescribes tablets.

Comment

Derek has managed to reduce the frequency of attacks by treating the cause—in his case, neck pain. Most attacks respond to simple treatment. Attacks on waking are typically more severe as symptoms have built up while the patient is asleep and cannot be treated early. Oral triptans can be considered. Subcutaneous or intranasal triptans are recommended if the patient is nauseous or vomiting. Analgesic and antiemetic suppositories are also useful in these circumstances or if triptans are contraindicated.

Case study

Claire, aged 22 and in her final year at university, studying English Literature was diagnosed as having migraine with aura. She has had several upsets recently which her doctor thought could account for the change in the attacks. She had not bothered to take medication for attacks as she felt nauseous. In addition to counselling about possible trigger factors, her doctor advises her to try a combination of an oral analgesic with domperidone as soon as she notices an aura starting. This means she will be taking medication before she feels too sick, and so may help treat the headache phase of the attack, although it would be unlikely to affect the aura symptoms. She is also given analgesic and antiemetic suppositories to use if nausea prohibits oral medication. Claire is very relieved to know that she has not got a brain tumour and that she also has something to control the symptoms. But she is still worried about the effect of migraine on her exam performance if these strategies are ineffective. The doctor considers the options. Final exams are not for several months, so a course of preventative treatment could be started in good time so that most side-effects will have worn off long before exams start. Propranolol is the obvious choice, but amitriptyline is an option. Claire is not keen to take medication daily. She asks about other treatments to take in the attack. The doctor discusses the new triptans which she could try and the different delivery methods. Claire feels reassured that additional treatments are available if she needs them. She promises to keep a record of her attacks and makes an appointment for review in a few weeks' time.

Comment

Claire's main problem is a fear of having a brain tumour. Reassurance may be all she needs but there are several possible approaches that the doctor has discussed. If Claire returns needing triptans, specific advice is necessary. There is evidence to show that triptans have limited effect if taken before the headache develops, so Claire should continue taking the analgesic/antiemetic combination at the onset of aura. She should take the triptan only as the headache develops. Headache recurs in about one-third of cases following triptan use. This is usually the following day, but can be later the same day. Treatment of recurrence should be appropriate to the severity of symptoms.

References

1 Tfelt-Hansen P, Henry P, Mulder K *et al.* The effectiveness of combined oral lysine acetylsalicylate and metoclopramide compared with oral sumatriptan for migraine. *Lancet* 1995; 346: 923–6.

2 Abd-El-Maeboud KH, El-Naggar T, El-Hawi EMM, Mahmoud SAR, Abd-El-Hay S. Rectal suppository: commonsense and mode of insertion. *Lancet* 1991; 338: 798–800.

3 Ottervanger JP, Stricker BHCh. Cardiovascular adverse reactions to sumatriptan: cause for concern? *CNS Drugs* 1995; 3: 90–8.

4 Ramadan NM, Schultz LL, Gilkey SJ. Migraine prophylactic drugs: proof of efficacy, utilization and cost. *Cephalalgia* 1997; 17: 73–80.

5 Mulleners WM, Whitmarsh TE, Steiner TJ. Noncompliance may render migraine prophylaxis useless, but once-daily regimens are better. *Cephalalgia* 1998; 18: 52–6.

6 Consumer Association. Prescribing unlicensed drugs or using drugs for unlicensed indications. *Drugs Ther Bull* 1992; 30: 97–9.

7 Hesse J, Mogelvang B, Simonsen H. Acupuncture versus metoprolol in migraine prophylaxis: a randomised trial of trigger point inactivation. *J Intern Med* 1994; 235: 451–6.

8 Holroyd KA, Penzien DB. Pharmacological versus non-pharmacological prophylaxis of recurrent migraine headache: a meta-analytic review of clinical trials. *Pain* 1990; 42 (1): 1–13.

9 Whitmarsh TE, Coleston-Shields DM, Steiner TJ. Double-blind randomised placebo-controlled study of homeopathic prophylaxis of migraine. *Cephalalgia* 1997; 17: 600–4.

8

CHAPTER 9

Improving Management

Targeting care is a necessary aspect of management as no doctor wishes to increase an already overstretched workload (Table 9.1). Fortunately for the GP, not every patient with migraine on their list needs to see a doctor, managing adequately with treatment from the pharmacist (Fig. 9.1). However, studies show that there is a group of patients with frequent attacks for whom simple analgesics are ineffective. This can result in significant disability with time lost from work and leisure activities. It is this group of patients who would most benefit from medical advice.

Identifying migraine

The GP is faced with two major issues: firstly, correct diagnosis of migraine, differentiating migraine from other headaches; secondly, creating an effective management strategy to include self-help approaches in addition to providing optimal drug therapy, as indicated.

Why patients lapse from care

Many of those who have sought medical advice for migraine subsequently stop consulting. The obvious reason is that the migraine has improved—the period of exacerbation is over, at least for the time be-

Table 9.1 Problems for GPs.

Limited education
At undergraduate and postgraduate levels
Diagnostic uncertainty
Careful history-taking essential
No diagnostic investigations available
Patient may have more than one headache
Fear of brain tumour etc.
False expectations of patients
Want a 'cure'
Want a 'brain scan'
Lack of time

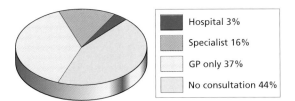

■	Hospital 3%
▨	Specialist 16%
□	GP only 37%
□	No consultation 44%

Fig. 9.1 Consultation rates. Based on data from Rasmussen BK. Epidemiology of headache. *Cephalalgia* 1995; 15: 45–68.

ing, or attacks are adequately controlled with over-the-counter therapy. But other reasons given include the belief that medication would not work based on dissatisfaction with previous treatments, failure of the patient to reach a shared understanding with their GP about the nature of the problem and what can reasonably be done to control symptoms, the feeling that the doctor does not consider migraine to be an important problem, or the belief that the doctor has little understanding or knowledge about migraine (Table 9.2).

It is not surprising that patients are far more satisfied with care that they receive from doctors who have migraine themselves than those who do not. This is not to say that all doctors must experience the illnesses that plague their patients in order to empathize with them but it does mean that gaining more understanding about the nature of the condition may improve care.

Improving the migraine consultation (Table 9.3)

Studies have shown that although doctors believe their patients want

Table 9.2 Why don't migraineurs consult?

They do not know it's migraine
Migraine not a problem
Infrequent attacks
Respond to over-the-counter therapy
'It's all in the mind'
Social stigma
'No effective treatment available'
Poor response to past treatment
Lack of management strategy
Incorrect diagnosis of migraine
Additional headaches
Unsupportive primary-care physician

effective drugs, patients actually put the need for an explanation of the cause of their pain higher on the list [1]. They also want an explanation about how medication works and possible side-effects—something which doctors in the studies failed to mention at all. This mismatch of needs can easily be overcome by improved consultation skills [2]. For example:

• Allow adequate time for the consultation and have an empathetic approach. Is it possible to conduct an adequate consultation within the time available or is more time needed?
• Confirm the diagnosis: history, examination and investigation.
• Ask about beliefs and fears; explain and reassure when appropriate.
• Consider the patients' expectations and develop a management strategy, explaining decisions made and offering different solutions where appropriate.
• Consider referral where appropriate.

Making a diagnosis is the most important initial step as incorrect diagnosis results in ineffective management. Perhaps the most common problem in making the diagnosis is the presence of more than one type of headache (Fig. 9.2). A careful history, examination, and the use of diary cards usually provides the answers. Unless the nature of the headache is obvious, it may be necessary to defer making the diagnosis until diary cards have been completed for a few weeks.

Management strategies can be targeted to the needs of the individual, as discussed in Chapter 8. An empathetic approach, listening to fears, providing a diagnosis and reassuring the patient that there is no sinister

Table 9.3 Improving management.

Provide time and empathy
Make a diagnosis
History
Examination
(Investigation)*
Offer reassurance
Explanation
Time for questions
Management strategy
Provide literature
Provide follow-up
Involve relative
Provide contact number
Involve other healthcare workers—practice nurse/physiotherapist
(Referral)*

*If indicated

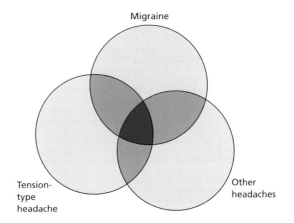

Fig. 9.2 Headaches can coexist.

underlying pathology are therapeutic measures in themselves that are often forgotten. Be realistic: do not promise a cure! The majority of patients are content to minimize the impact of migraine on home and working life. Confront patient expectations: many patients may wonder why they have not been prescribed the new 'wonder' drug mentioned in a magazine they have read, or may feel that they should be

Table 9.4 Management in general practice: new cases.

Accurate diagnosis	History, examination and use of diary cards
Initiate management strategy	Reassurance and discussion of patient's concerns
	Non-drug strategies for prevention and consideration of options for drug therapy, acute ± prophylactic
	Make follow-up appointment
Refer to practice nurse/ nurse practitioner	Counselling and provision of information for patient and family. Instruction in diary cards and use of medication
Refer to other healthcare workers, e.g. physiotherapist/counsellor	Treatment of muscle contraction/ teaching coping strategies
Refer to patient association	Provision of further information and support: see Appendix A
Refer to specialist	If evidence of underlying pathology

Table 9.5 Management in general practice: review.

Check

Review of diary cards

Diagnosis: is it migraine? Are there additional headaches?

Frequency, duration and type of migraine

Compliance, efficacy and side-effects of medication

Continuing education/information

Patient fears, effect of migraine on life

Changing circumstances: effect on new job, change of contraception, pregnancy, etc.

Follow-up appointment

Consider intervention

Medication requires adjustment: adjust acute therapy, initiate prophylaxis

Consider stopping prophylaxis if attacks under control

Consider referral to specialist

Diagnostic uncertainty

Treatment failure

Patient request

Onset of new symptoms suggestive of underlying pathology

For advice on special circumstances—migraine in children, hormonal triggers, etc.

Consideration of new drugs/treatment options

9

sent for a brain scan. It is also worthwhile explaining that a trial of different treatments may be necessary before the most effective is found.

Consultations for a first visit for migraine and the follow-up visits require a different emphasis (Tables 9.4 & 9.5).

The need for information and counselling

Although migraine is now recognized as an organic condition, it still carries a stigma of people who are 'unable to cope' or 'unreliable'. A study of members attending a Migraine Action Association meeting revealed that 73% of the audience considered that there was a social stigma associated with migraine and that migraine was not a condition that many non-sufferers took seriously. It is now recognized that migraine can be associated with significant disability, affecting relationships with friends, family and employers. This is made worse by the added impact that frequent attacks can have due to time lost from work and leisure activities. It follows that it is not only the patient who needs information: involving family and providing literature to take to employers can remove some of the burden of coping with migraine. If the public understand that migraine is more than 'just a headache', those with migraine are more able to address migraine as a problem and integrate it into their lives. A better understanding of the true nature of migraine may help identify those labelled as having 'refractory' migraine who actually have different or additional headaches requiring specific treatment.

Using a checklist

It is useful to have a structure to follow to ensure that important basic information is not overlooked (Table 9.6). The aim is to provide the

Table 9.6 Information checklist.

About migraine	Lifestyle implications
What migraine is	Employment
What happens during an attack	Social life
Treatments available (drug and non-drug)	Contraception (only migraine with aura)
Prognosis	
	About drugs
Precipitating factors	Acute and prophylactic options
Insufficient food	How they work
Certain foods	How to take them
Strenuous exercise	Side-effects
Hormonal fluctuations	Duration of prophylactic therapy
Illness	
Musculoskeletal pain	Support groups
Changes in sleep patterns	Migraine Action Association
Stress	Migraine Trust
Travel	
Weather	Sources of literature
Emotional upsets	Library
	Support groups
	Pharmaceutical companies

information necessary for patients which will enable them to help themselves. Listening carefully is also important. Many patients attending a specialist clinic remark how much it helps to have someone take them seriously and who will listen to their problems. Unfortunately, providing this type of service takes time but time invested in the early consultations makes future consultations less likely. How can this be achieved without adding an additional burden to an already overworked GP? The usual consultation time available to most GPs will be insufficient. Although the diagnosis can usually be made within the first few minutes, additional time is necessary to listen to the patient, undertake the examination, reassure, discuss management strategies and answer any questions. This takes even longer if a friend or relative is present. Delegating to other healthcare workers or providing contact addresses of support groups can reduce the time spent by the doctor. Suggested answers to the questions are given in Chapter 16. Triggers are covered in more detail in Chapters 6 and 8. Information on support groups is listed in Appendix A. Few people take in everything that is said in any consultation and it helps to have supporting literature for them to take home.

Involving other healthcare professionals

Practice nurse/nurse practitioner

Once the diagnosis has been made, there are several management issues that can be undertaken by trained practice nurse/nurse practitioners. Patients often feel more comfortable with nursing staff as they perceive that they have more time to listen and there is less of a professional 'barrier'. This puts the practice nurse/nurse practitioner in a useful liaison position between doctor and patient.

Explanation

The practice nurse/nurse practitioner can make sure that the patient understands and agrees with the information and advice given by the GP. Educational literature about migraine can be provided, together with a simple explanation of the nature of the condition, prognosis and treatments available. The latter should include non-drug as well as drug options.

Advice on trigger factors and diary cards is given in Chapter 8.

How to optimize drug therapy

Although the doctor may have provided a prescription for an effective drug, there are simple ways to improve efficacy further. Patients should be instructed at what stage of an attack they should take drugs, likely side-effects and what to do if treatment fails. Advice on prophylactic drugs should include the need to take drugs at regular intervals.

Continuing care

Patients can be given a contact number in case of problems. It is surprising how few patients will use this if it is given to them. The nurse can also ensure that a follow-up appointment has been made. In particular, this is necessary in order to assess diaries as well as the effectiveness of management strategies.

Counsellors

An increasing number of clinics have access to counselling services. This can be very useful if there are underlying issues such as family concerns, work difficulties or underlying depression related to events.

Physiotherapists

This is also an increasing service in primary care. Muscle contraction is a common cause of headache and may accompany migraine, therefore physiotherapy can be useful for headache management. Drug therapy is best avoided as it only treats symptoms, not the cause. Patients can be taught simple exercises to loosen tense muscles and be instructed how to avoid developing further muscle problems in their daily activities. This may seem an expensive strategy initially but it is more likely to result in long-term relief.

When to refer

Migraine is a condition that can be managed effectively in primary care. Consequently, fewer than 5% of cases are referred. But there are times when referral is indicated and it is not only patients with suspected underlying pathology who benefit from specialist care. Research has shown that the experience of a hospital referral can have significant therapeutic influence, independent of treatment offered. This is particularly beneficial when simple management strategies prove ineffec-

9

tive or when a patient is not convinced of the diagnosis given. The most common reasons for referral include concern about diagnosis, treatment failure and patient request [3].

Some of these referrals could be avoided. Failure of treatment response is often due to failure to recognize the presence of an additional headache, which could have been identified by a more thorough history.

An increasing number of migraine clinics are opening, usually on a sessional basis attached to an NHS neurology department. A few clinics are full-time and, if run as charities, may not charge referring GPs. Some clinics have a specialist interest in children or the effects of hormones on headache and can offer advice on particular management problems. Further information on clinics can be found in Appendix A.

Writing a referral letter

The information included in the referral letter is invaluable to the specialist. Unfortunately, the information provided is often inadequate. It is not necessary to write a long letter but it is helpful to include:

- provisional diagnosis;
- current drug therapy, including doses and duration of use;
- past drug therapy, including doses and duration of use, and sensitivities;
- investigations and outcome;
- other management strategies tried;
- any previous referrals and outcome;
- other medical or psychiatric problems;
- reason for referral, for example help with diagnosis, advice on a specific course of treatment, or even at the patient's request.

This information can save a great deal of the specialist's time and may avoid repetition of previously tried management strategies.

Developing a protocol for integrated care

Protocols are useful in clinical practice, providing a structure for delegation of responsibility between the doctor and other healthcare workers, typically the practice nurse/nurse practitioner.

Such a protocol should cover the following aspects.
- Aims and objectives of the service.
- Staff requirements to run the service, including training.
- Time requirements per session and per patient.
- Referral system: to the practice nurse/nurse practitioner and from the practice nurse/nurse practitioner to others.

9

- Duties: including information to be obtained from the patient and information to be provided by the nurse, for example instruction in the completion of diary cards and subsequent review.
- Treatment details: in some cases the doctor may delegate the responsibility of administration of a prescription-only medicine. This is regulated by the Medicines Act 1968. Section 58 (2) (b) states that a person may administer a prescription-only medicine in accordance with the directions of an appropriate practitioner. The Act defines the 'appropriate practitioner' as a doctor but 'direction' is open to broader interpretation. A written protocol provides documentary evidence that 'direction' has been provided by the doctor to enable the nurse to prescribe in accordance with the Act.
- Documentation: records of patient care are legal documents and should be retained for a minimum of 10 years. Information should be accurately recorded, signed and dated.
- Emergency procedure: how the nurse will request medical back-up.
- Evaluation and audit: continuing review of the success of the service is necessary with subsequent updating of protocols.

Avoiding medico-legal headaches

Fear of litigation is an increasing problem for all doctors. The unfortunate outcome can be the adoption of defensive practice that, in the case of headache can, for example, result in unnecessary investigations for fear of missing tumours. Overuse of investigations can increase patient morbidity.

There are two main reasons for litigation. First, misdiagnosis. Examples include: a patient with phaeochromocytoma diagnosed as migraine who subsequently developed a stroke; or the patient whose transient ischaemic attacks were diagnosed as migraine aura and who also subsequently developed a stroke. Secondly, failure to warn of the danger of drugs and possible side-effects. An example of this is a woman given sodium valproate for migraine prophylaxis who was not warned about the need for adequate contraception. It was not until she became pregnant that she discovered the high incidence of fetal abnormalities associated with use of sodium valproate. On a lighter note is the patient, having been advised to use a pack of frozen peas to relieve muscle tension, was not advised to wrap a cloth around it. She developed frostbite!

All patients went on to successfully sue the doctor. All these situations could have been avoided if good medical practice had been followed.

The courts have usually applied the standard of the reasonable professional exercising a particular skill to determine liability. This is known as the 'Bolam' standard, outlined by Lord Scarman in his speech following the House of Lords decision of Sidaway vs. Bethlem Royal Hospital. If there is a body of competent professional opinion that supports the defendant's actions, a claim for negligence will fail. The standards applied are those that were acceptable at the time of the alleged negligence. However, this is not always applied in practice and cannot be relied upon as a line of defence. Advice should be sought from the appropriate medical defence organization.

Several other points are worthy of note.
• Pay careful attention to obtaining patients' consent and providing warnings of risk.
• Keep meticulous records, documenting discussion of risks.
• Tasks delegated to other staff should be properly supervised and follow an agreed protocol.
• Complaints should be handled quickly, by senior staff. Patients may feel angry and bitter, feelings that can be abated by careful handling.

Why patients sue

Studies show that intense negative emotion plays a significant part in the decision by patients to take legal action. Four main reasons for litigation have been identified.
1   Concerns with standards of care—the wish to prevent similar incidents in the future.
2   The need for an explanation—to know how the injury happened and why.
3   Compensation—for actual losses, pain and suffering or to provide future care for the injured party.
4   Accountability—a belief that the staff involved should take account for their actions.

It follows that time spent investigating a complaint at the outset could prevent the complaint going further. It is important to make sure that each point a complainant makes is dealt with fully. Even seemingly trivial issues should be taken seriously as they can indicate a breakdown in communication. Most Health Authorities have a practice-based response to complaints. One member of the practice team, usually the practice manager, is responsible for managing all complaints in an impartial way. This includes logging the complaint, interviewing the patient to discover the exact nature of the complaint, investigating the issues raised and reporting back to the patient. Whilst this open method may result in more complaints coming to the attention of the partners, it is likely that the vast majority can be dealt with in the practice, with fewer complaints referred to the Health Authority. A careful written response or a face-to-face meeting with the patient can avert further action, provided an acrimonious confrontation can be avoided. It is important to inform the complainant how the matter was investigated and what changes have been made as a result of the complaint. At least 75% of complaints can satisfactorily be resolved in this way [4].

Patients who remain dissatisfied may approach the Health Authority with a request for independent review.

References

1 Packard RC. What does the headache patient want? *Headache* 1979; 19: 370–4.
2 MacGregor EA. The doctor and the migraine patient: improving compliance. *Neurology* 1997; 48 (Suppl. 3): S16–20.
3 Blau JN, MacGregor EA. Migraine consultations: a triangle of view points. *Headache* 1995; 35: 104–6.
4 Bingham E. The ombudsman and general practice. *J MDU* 1998; 14: 6–8.

9

CHAPTER 10

Hormonal Headaches

Empirical evidence supports a hormonal trigger for migraine although the true role of hormones is complex and not fully understood. Until puberty, migraine is equally common in boys and girls with increasing female predominance following menarche. During the reproductive years, migraine becomes three times more common in women than in men. The effect of hormones on migraine is greater for migraine without aura than for migraine with aura, even in women who have both types of attacks.

Migraine associated with menstruation

At least 50% of female migraineurs report an association between migraine and menstruation. However, fewer than 10% of women have attacks that link to possible specific, and treatable, hormonal mechanisms.

Certainly, menstruation is a time of increased likelihood of migraine but for most of these women the association is inconsistent, or they have several attacks throughout the cycle (Fig. 10.1). In such women, hormonal triggers are likely to be additional to non-hormonal triggers. This is important for management as hormonal treatment may not be effective. Management of the non-hormonal factors is more appropriate in the first instance.

True 'menstrual' migraine has been defined as 'attacks of migraine without aura that occur regularly on day 1 of menstruation ± 2 days and at no other time' [1].

Correct diagnosis is essential for successful management and specific treatments should not be instigated until the diagnosis has been confirmed by diary card evidence. Of the two major hormones produced by the ovaries during the menstrual cycle, clinical and scientific studies show that the natural fall in oestrogen before menstruation, and not the fall in progesterone, is a trigger for migraine in some susceptible women (Figs 10.2 & 10.3) [2]. But sex hormones are not solely responsible, as some women are sensitive to other events, for example prostaglandin release during menstruation. No specific tests are currently available to confirm the diagnosis as studies show that there are no

10

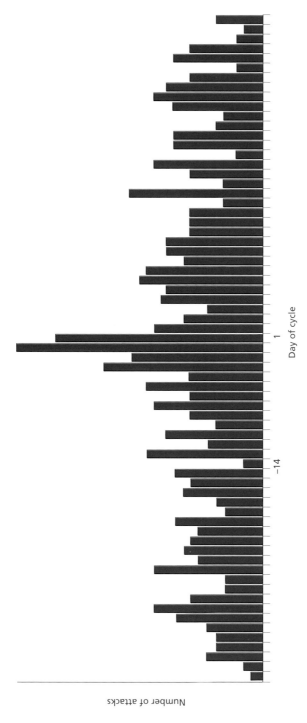

Fig. 10.1 The peak frequency of migraine in 55 women over three menstrual cycles. Day 1 = first day of bleeding; day –14 = ovulation. Reproduced with permission from MacGregor EA. "Menstrual" migraine: towards a definition. *Cephalalgia* 1996; 16: 11–21.

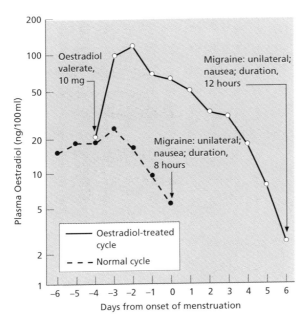

Fig. 10.2 The effect of treatment with oestradiol valerate upon menstrual migraine. Reproduced with permission from Somerville BW. The role of estradiol withdrawal in the etiology of menstrual migraine. *Neurology* 1972; 22: 358.

10

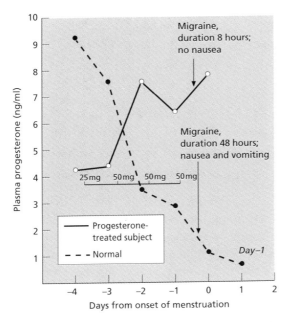

Fig. 10.3 The effect of treatment with progesterone upon menstrual migraine. Reproduced with permission from Somerville BW. The role of progesterone in menstrual migraine. *Neurology* 1971; 21: 855.

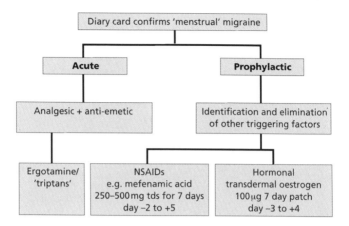

Fig. 10.4 Management of 'menstrual' migraine.

measurable differences in hormone levels in women with menstrual migraine, compared with control groups. It would appear that these women are more sensitive to the effects of normal fluctuations.

Management of 'menstrual' migraine (Fig. 10.4)

The following recommendations for management are for menstruating women who are not using any hormonal therapy. The associations between migraine and hormonal contraception or replacement therapy are separate issues, discussed below.

When a woman presents with a possible hormonal trigger, it is necessary first to confirm the diagnosis of migraine by history and examination, and then to confirm the hormonal link with diary cards.

Diary cards

Simple diary cards (Fig. 10.5) can be used to confirm or refute an association of migraine with menstruation. They can also highlight menstrual irregularities and be used to record associated premenstrual or menopausal symptoms. Women should be asked to complete the diary cards as accurately as possible. Records should be kept for a minimum of 3 months. During this time, attack therapy can be discussed and optimized. Ideally, women should also keep a trigger diary in order to identify potential non-hormonal triggers, as management of these can reduce the impact of hormonal triggers.

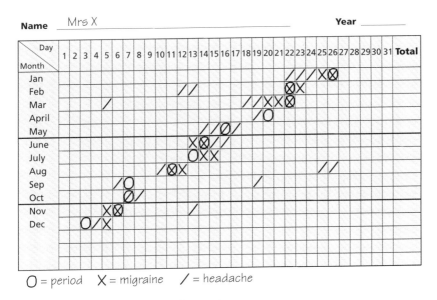

Name Mrs X   **Year** _____

Day / Month	1	2	3	4	5	6	7	8	9	10	11	12	13	14	15	16	17	18	19	20	21	22	23	24	25	26	27	28	29	30	31	**Total**
Jan																							/	/	/	X	⊗					
Feb												/	/								⊗	X										
Mar				/													/	/	X	X	⊗											
April																		/	O													
May													/	/	/	O	/															
June													X	⊗	/	/																
July													O	X	X																	
Aug											/	⊗	X											/	/							
Sep					/	O												/														
Oct						∅	/																									
Nov				X	⊗							/																				
Dec		O	/	X																												

O = period   X = migraine   / = headache

Fig. 10.5 Diary card of 'menstrual' migraine.

Attack therapy

Effective attack therapy may be all that is required if attacks are only occurring once a month. Standard acute treatments are recommended. However, there is some evidence that attacks linked to menstruation are less responsive to treatment, and recurrence of symptoms more likely to occur, compared with attacks occurring at other times of the menstrual cycle. One possible reason for this is the longer duration of the 'menstrual' trigger.

Prophylaxis

By the time that the diary cards are reviewed at follow-up, a percentage of patients will have their attacks under control without the need for further intervention. Another group will have attacks throughout the cycle, which are not obviously related to menstruation. These women may benefit from standard prophylactic therapy, if considered necessary.

Only a small percentage of women will have attacks of 'menstrual' migraine, as defined above, requiring specific prophylaxis. Depending on each woman's wishes, and need for contraception, several options can be tried, both non-hormonal and hormonal. Prophylaxis should be tried for a minimum of three cycles, increasing to maximum dose, before being deemed ineffective. No drug is universally effective or tolerated, therefore each regimen should be tailored to the individual patient.

Non-hormonal prophylaxis

Many hormonal regimens depend on regular menstruation. Non-hormonal prophylaxis can be effective when taken at the onset of bleeding. This is a particular advantage for women with erratic cycles. Non-steroidal anti-inflammatory drugs (NSAIDs) would appear to be the most effective prophylactic used in this way. The mechanism of action of these drugs is unknown but may be related to perimenstrual prostaglandin release from the uterus, maximal on the first day of bleeding.

Mefenamic acid is probably the drug of choice, 500 mg three to four times daily. This should be started either 2–3 days before the expected onset of menstruation, or started on the first day of bleeding. It is particularly helpful in reducing associated menorrhagia and/or dysmenorrhoea.

Some studies have suggested **Naproxen** 550 mg once or twice daily from 7 days before menstruation for a total of 14 days.

Alternatively, **Fenoprofen** 600 mg can be taken twice daily from 3 days before the onset of menstruation until the last day of bleeding.

Hormonal prophylaxis

If non-hormonal treatments are ineffective, a trial of hormonal intervention can be considered.

Perimenstrual. Unless a woman also needs contraception, perimenstrual oestrogen supplements can be used to prevent the natural oestrogen drop in the late luteal phase of the menstrual cycle. Although this regimen uses treatments normally given for hormone replacement therapy, it is important to note that for 'menstrual' migraine, hormones are given as supplements. This means that if the woman has an intact uterus, and provided she is ovulating regularly, no additional progestogens are necessary. This is because she will be producing adequate amounts of her own natural progesterone to counter the effects of unopposed oestrogen, which could otherwise lead to endometrial proliferation. Ovulation can be confirmed, if necessary, with blood levels of progesterone taken 7 days before expected menstruation, i.e. day 21 of a 28-day cycle. The level should be greater than 30 nmol/l.

Transdermal oestrogen 100 µg can be used from approximately 3 days before expected menstruation for about 7 days, i.e. two twice-weekly patches or one 7-day patch. If this regimen is effective but side-effects are a problem (bloating, breast tenderness, leg cramps, nausea) a 50-µg dose should be tried for the next cycle.

Alternatively, **oestradiol gel 1.5 mg in 2.5 g gel** can be applied daily from 3 days before expected menstruation for 7 days. This regimen may be more effective than transdermal patches as the gel produces higher, more stable, levels of oestrogen. However, it is less convenient for most women than the 7-day patches.

Oestrogen supplements should not be used by women who are at risk of pregnancy, have undiagnosed vaginal bleeding, or oestrogen-dependent tumours such as those affecting the breast or endometrium.

Continuous. Most of these regimens also have the advantage of a contraceptive action.

Combined oral contraception (COC) inhibits ovulation, producing fairly stable oestrogen levels when taken, and can improve migraine in some women. The pill-free interval is associated with a drop in the level of oestrogen which can trigger migraine, similar to the trigger for 'menstrual' migraine. Although COCs are safe for the majority of women, certain groups of women are recommended to use COCs with caution, or to use alternative contraception. Standard COC prescribing recommendations should be followed [3]. Recommendations relating to use of COCs in women with migraine are given below.

Levonorgestrel (Mirena®) Intra-uterine System (IUS) is licensed for contraception but is also highly effective at reducing menstrual bleeding and associated pain. It appears to be effective in migraine that is related to dysmenorrhoea and/or menorrhagia. It is not effective for women who are sensitive to oestrogen withdrawal as a migraine trigger, as the majority of women still ovulate with the system *in situ*. Its mode of action is to release progestogen directly to the uterus, preventing the endometrial response to oestrogen and creating thickened cervical mucus inhibiting the transport of sperm. Systemic effects are usually minor but erratic bleeding and spotting is common in the early months of use. However, most women are amenorrhoeic at 1 year. It is most likely to help women whose 'menstrual' migraine responds to prostaglandin inhibitors, for example mefenamic acid, particularly if they also require contraception. Oestrogen supplements can be given if climacteric symptoms develop, without the need for additional progestogens. However, at the time of writing, the IUS is not licensed for hormone replacement therapy (HRT).

10

Injectable depot progestogens provide highly effective contraception by inhibiting ovulation, similar to the mode of action of COCs. Although irregular bleeding can occur in early months of treatment, this method has the advantage that in most cases menstruation ceases. By inhibiting the normal menstrual cycle, hormonal triggers are removed. A few women appear to be sensitive to progestogens, developing premenstrual-type symptoms, although this is less likely with progesterone derivatives such as medroxyprogesterone acetate, than with testosterone derivatives such as norethisterone.

Oral progestogen-only contraception does not inhibit ovulation, is associated with a disrupted menstrual cycle, and therefore has little place in the management of 'menstrual' migraine.

Gonadotrophin-releasing hormones have been tried but climacteric side-effects, for example hot flushes, restrict their use. They are also associated with a marked reduction in bone density and should not usually be used regularly for longer than 6 months without regular monitoring and bone densitometry. Add-back continuous oestrogen and progestogen can be given to counter these difficulties. Given these limitations, in addition to increased cost, such treatment is best instigated in specialist departments.

Hysterectomy has no place in the management of migraine alone. Studies show that migraine is more likely to deteriorate after surgical menopause with bilateral oophorectomy. Even if an oophorectomy is not performed, hysterectomy often precipitates an early menopause. However, if other medical problems necessitate surgical menopause, the effects may be lessened by subsequent oestrogen replacement therapy.

Case study

Linda is 38 and has a full-time office job. She had her first migraine when she was 36 and currently has two attacks per month. Each attack lasts up to 2 days and she is free from symptoms between attacks. She feels that they are related to her menstrual cycle but this was not confirmed by diary card. The attacks either start early evening or are present on waking. Her eyes feel tired and she finds herself squinting. She then develops a right- or left-sided headache associated with anorexia, nausea, vomiting, dysphasia, dizziness, photophobia, phonophobia and osmophobia. She has to stay in bed for most of the 2 days and it takes a further day before she feels back to normal. The doctor diagnosed migraine without aura and has tried numerous acute treatments, including oral and intranasal sumatriptan, without success. Examina-

tion was normal, with the exception of elevated blood pressure, which has been 140/95 at each of the last three visits.

The doctor discusses management options with Linda. Linda agrees that the diary confirms that there is no clear link with menstruation but is unhappy that she has not found an effective means of controlling symptoms. The doctor suggests a trial of prophylactic medication. Linda agrees, leaving the surgery with a prescription for propranolol. When she returns for review a couple of months later, she has only had one severe attack, which was shortly after she started treatment. She says she felt attacks developing on a couple of occasions, but symptoms responded to simple analgesics.

Comment

Although acute medication is all that is usually necessary for management of two migraine attacks per month, the problem is how to treat attacks that do not respond. Diary cards were helpful in confirming that there was no true menstrual link, so hormonal therapies are not appropriate. Since Linda has slightly raised blood pressure, it may be to her advantage to try β-blockers for prophylaxis. She will need to continue this for 4–6 months, with regular checks of blood pressure during and after cessation of treatment. Although hypertension is rarely a cause of headache, it will still need to be managed if it remains high. Simple strategies, such as weight loss and smoking cessation, may help but β-blockers could be continued, if necessary.

10

Case study

Audrey is 43. She had her first migraine at the age of 19, around the same time as she started the combined oral contraceptive pill. At that time she had one or two attacks a year, usually at times of stress. She became pregnant with her first child when she was 31 and, although she had several attacks in the early months of pregnancy, she was then free of migraine for 7 years. The attacks returned about 1 year after the birth of her second child. At first they were infrequent and were more likely to occur at weekends or when she was overtired. As the migraines became more frequent, she noticed that they would often start on the first or second day of her period. Her periods were regular but had become quite heavy and painful. She took ibuprofen to ease the period pains, and to treat migraine. She describes symptoms typical of migraine without aura. Most last about 3 days. She is free from symptoms between attacks. Audrey presents to her doctor for help with *'menstrual' migraines. The doctor asks Audrey to keep a record of her symptoms and recommends an analgesic/antiemetic for acute treatment. At her follow-up appointment, Audrey's diary cards confirm 'menstrual' migraine. The doctor recommends mefenamic acid, 500 mg three to four times daily for 5 days from the start of bleeding, since this usually preceded the onset of migraine. Audrey had found that the analgesic/antiemetic preparation took the edge off the migraine but did not control it completely. The doctor suggests that Audrey perseveres for the next couple of cycles as the mefenamic acid might control symptoms. Audrey makes another appointment to see the doctor in a couple of months to discuss the need for any further changes in treatment.*

Comment

Audrey has 'menstrual' migraine associated with heavy, painful periods. A prostaglandin inhibitor can be used to control both symptoms. Prophylaxis can make attacks more responsive to acute treatment, so the doctor was right not to change acute treatment immediately until the effects of prophylaxis could be assessed. If more effective treatment were required, a triptan would probably be the drug of choice. However, recurrence of symptoms for several consecutive days is not uncommon in migraine linked to menstruation. In these situations, treatment with ergotamine or dihydroergotamine may be more effective as these drugs have a longer duration of action. Nausea is a common side-effect which can be controlled with concomitant domperidone or metoclopramide. If Audrey did not have problems with her periods, it would still be worthwhile trying a prostaglandin inhibitor as a first-line prophylactic. If this is not effective, further recommendations depend on the need for contraception and the regularity of menstruation. Audrey does not need contraception as her husband has been sterilized and her periods are regular, so she could try perimenstrual oestrogen supplements if she wished.

Migraine associated with the premenstrual syndrome

A percentage of women are more prone to attacks of migraine premenstrually, often in association with other premenstrual symptoms.

Diagnosis of all symptoms can be confirmed with diary cards, which should show a pattern of symptoms only during the second half of the menstrual cycle, relieved by menstruation.

Management of premenstrual migraine

Non-drug management

The premenstrual syndrome is identified by diary card evidence, kept for at least 3 months, since no tests are available to confirm the diagnosis. In addition to migraine, symptoms include abdominal distension, malaise, cyclical mastalgia, irritability, depression and aggression.

Many women benefit from simple non-drug strategies for management including relaxation, psychotherapy, acupuncture and yoga. General health advice to take regular exercise and eat frequent carbohydrate snacks may help—there is evidence that some women experience impaired glucose tolerance curve at this stage of the menstrual cycle.

Drug management

Non-hormonal

Many drugs have been used for the treatment of premenstrual symptoms but few have been shown to be effective. This is particularly the case for **pyridoxine (vitamin B6)** which, although widely advocated, has limited value for this condition. There has been concern about the high dose vitamin B6 and over-the-counter doses are restricted. Doses over 500 mg/day have been associated with peripheral neuropathy. Indigestion and gastritis have also been reported in doses over 100 mg/day. Women wishing to try vitamin B6 are recommended to start with 50 mg once or twice daily and should not exceed 200 mg/day. This should be started about 10–14 days before the expected onset of menses but may be taken continuously if cycles are irregular.

Oil of evening primrose containing gamolenic acid is certainly effective for cyclical mastalgia in doses of 120–160 mg twice daily.

More recently, trials using **selective serotonin re-uptake inhibitors**, for example fluoxetine (20 mg/day), have shown encouraging results. Concomitant use of sumatriptan is contraindicated.

Hormonal

Hormonal treatments for premenstrual symptoms are used to alter or eliminate the natural ovarian cycle. If menstruation is regular, **oestrogen supplements** can be given as for 'menstrual' migraine but in a lower dose of 25 µg every 3–4 days. This should be started 7–10 days before

10

the expected onset of menstruation and stopped at the onset of bleeding.

Hormonal treatments that eliminate the ovarian cycle can also be tried for the management of premenstrual symptoms but there are little clinical data available on efficacy. These include **injectable depot progestogens** and **combined oral contraceptives**. **Gonadotrophin-releasing hormone agonists** are the most reliable means to suppress ovarian activity, inducing a 'reversible' menopause. Only short-term therapy is recommended, as discussed for 'menstrual' migraine.

Migraine and hormone replacement therapy

Migraine is a common problem in the perimenopause. In some cases this may result from increased stresses, depression and musculoskeletal problems that are more prominent at this time of life. These should respond to standard management strategies.

Women with menopausal symptoms, and exacerbation of migraine resulting from erratic oestrogen secretion, benefit from HRT. Optimal treatment stabilizes oestrogen fluctuations and can control migraine. Adequate, stable levels of oestrogen are necessary, best provided by percutaneous or transdermal methods used continuously. Hysterectomized women could consider oestrogen implants.

Headaches can be associated with cyclical progestogens, necessary for unhysterectomized women. Changing the type of progestogen is usually sufficient. Clinically, headache is less of a problem with progesterone derivatives including dydrogesterone or medroxyprogesterone acetate, than with testosterone derivatives such as norethisterone. Transdermal progestogens are another option. Alternatively, natural progesterone therapy could be considered. Postmenopausal women appear to have fewer problems with migraine when using continuous combined no-bleed regimens. These can be used by women 1 year after the natural menopause. Irregular bleeding is a common problem if this regimen is used earlier. Even postmenopausal women starting continuous combined replacement therapy may experience some bleeding in the earlier months of use but this usually settles within 6 months and does not usually warrant investigation.

Migraineurs experiencing severe hot flushes, who do not wish to take hormonal treatments, may benefit from **clonidine** prophylaxis. The dose is 50–75 μg twice daily. Side-effects include sedation, dry mouth, dizziness and insomnia. Clonidine was originally developed as an antihypertensive and consequently interacts with other antihypertensive drugs.

10

Case study

Audrey's 'menstrual' migraine attacks were kept under control for several years using a combination of acute treatments and prophylactic mefenamic acid. However, she is now 49 and is back in the surgery as her periods have become irregular and she is getting frequent hot flushes and night sweats. She still gets migraine with her periods but also has attacks at other times of the cycle. Consequently, she is having an attack about once every 10 days. Although she can control these with acute treatments, the frequency of attacks is getting her down and the night sweats are leaving her exhausted. She is losing time from work and worries that she might be made redundant. Her doctor discusses a trial of HRT to treat menopausal symptoms and regulate her periods. Audrey starts on transdermal cyclical HRT and makes an appointment for review in 3 months. When she returns, she reports to the doctor that the hot flushes and night sweats have settled. She has had two migraine attacks but these were most probably due to a busy time at work. Her periods seem to be settling and she is happy to continue the HRT. She makes an appointment for a check-up in a further 3 months' time.

10

Comment

The menopause marks a time of increased migraine. HRT can help migraine, particularly if disrupted sleep resulting from night sweats and mood swings due to hormone fluctuations become additional migraine triggers. HRT should only be started when periods become erratic and other menopausal symptoms are present. If HRT is started too early, side-effects from too much oestrogen are often a problem and can deter the woman from trying HRT at a more appropriate stage of the menopause. Non-oral routes of HRT are recommended for women with migraine as these provide the most stable levels of hormone.

Migraine and contraception

Combined oral contraceptives

Headache is a common side-effect of oral contraception. Many women report onset of migraine after starting COCs. Deterioration is not universal—many others report improvement of pre-existing migraine.

The concern is that both migraine and COCs are independent risk factors for stroke in young women, the latter related to the ethinyloestradiol component. Ischaemic stroke is rare in healthy women of reproductive age, with an annual incidence of approximately 2 per 100 000 at age 20, rising to 20 per 100 000 at age 40.

Use of COCs appears slightly to increase this risk, though it can be reduced if users are younger than 35 years, do not smoke, do not have a history of hypertension, and have normal blood pressure measured before starting COCs.

Migraine is associated with a relative risk for ischaemic stroke of between 2 and 3.7. Tzourio *et al.* found that migraine with aura was associated with twice the risk of ischaemic stroke than migraine without aura [4]. Use of COCs in women with migraine increased the odds ratio for ischaemic stroke to 13.9. The combination of heavy smoking (more than 20 cigarettes a day) and migraine was associated with an odds ratio of 10.2. Because of the small numbers involved in this study, it was not possible for the authors to assess other combined risk factors.

Although stroke in this age group is extremely rare, some caution is necessary when prescribing COCs to certain women with migraine, although it should be stressed that use of COCs is safe for the majority. Careful assessment of other risk factors, particularly smoking and hypertension, should be undertaken before and during COC use, in line with recommended prescribing practice [3]. Withdrawal of COCs should be considered if migraine or other headaches increase in frequency or severity with COC use (Table 10.1). Alternative methods of contraception, including progestogen-only methods, can be discussed. They should be offered to all women at risk, provided no other contraindications to their use apply.

The Faculty of Family Planning of the Royal College of Obstetricians and Gynaecologists have published the following recommendations for the use of COCs in migraineurs (Fig. 10.6) [5].

Table 10.1 Symptoms that may require discontinuation of the COC in women with pre-existing migraine without aura (if no other readily treatable cause is identified).

Change in migraine
Increased frequency of attacks
Increased duration of attacks
Increased severity of attacks
Development of focal symptoms
Change in non-migraine headaches
Increased severity
Increased frequency
Development of neurological symptoms, with or without headache

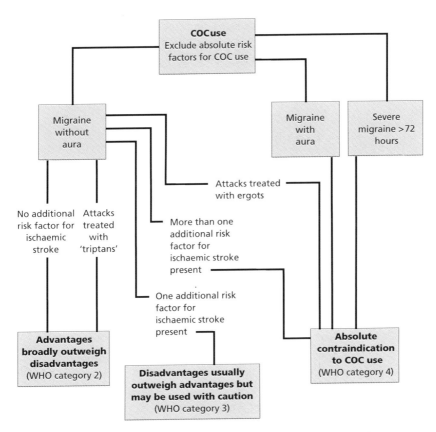

Fig. 10.6 The use of COCs in migraine. Reproduced from MacGregor EA, Guillebaud J. Recommendations for clinical practice: combined oral contraceptives, migraine and stroke. *Br J Fam Planning* 1998; 24: 53–60.

Situations where the advantages of COC use usually outweigh the disadvantages

- **Migraine without aura in the absence of additional risk factors for stroke**.
- **Triptan treatment**. Triptans (including sumatriptan, naratriptan and zolmitriptan) are selective vasoconstrictor drugs. They have been taken by many women using COCs and can be prescribed provided there are no contraindications to their use as specified in the data sheets.

Situations where the disadvantages of COC use usually outweigh the advantages

- **Migraine without aura in the presence of one additional risk factor for stroke**. Caution is indicated in women who have a history of one additional risk factor for stroke that is not, in itself, sufficiently severe to absolutely contraindicate COC use. Women should be counselled to reduce risk factors where appropriate, particularly smoking. COCs should be withdrawn if any further risk factor develops.

Absolute contraindications to COC use

• **Migraine with aura**. This recommendation is based on the increased risk of stroke in women having attacks with aura compared with women having attacks without aura. Focal symptoms of aura may indicate reduced cerebral blood flow which, coupled with the prothrombotic changes due to ethinyloestradiol, may be sufficient to tip the balance towards a thrombotic stroke. COCs should be discontinued immediately if any woman with a history of migraine without aura develops focal neurological symptoms. They can be transferred immediately, even during an attack, to the progestogen-only pill or other oestrogen-free contraception.

• **Migraine without aura in the presence of two or more additional risk factors for stroke**. COCs are not recommended for use in women who have multiple risk factors, whether or not these include migraine [3].

• **Severe migraine** ('status migrainosus'). COC use is also contraindicated for women who frequently have attacks of migraine which are unusually severe, or last longer than 72 h, despite treatment. The risk is related to the difficulty that can arise in distinguishing between migraine and organic cerebral ischaemia. If considered necessary, appropriate investigations should exclude underlying disease. The history should also exclude medication misuse, which can be associated with apparent increased frequency and severity of migraine.

• **Migraine treated with ergot derivatives**. Ergot alkaloids, including ergotamine and dihydroergotamine, have widespread vasoconstrictor actions. Their use has been associated with arterial thrombosis.

Migraine in the pill-free interval

Oestrogen levels fall during the pill-free week. Migraine occurring during this time appears to be triggered by oestrogen withdrawal, similar to the mechanism of 'menstrual' migraine. Effective acute treatment may be adequate. Failing this, the woman may try the 'tricycle' regimen, i.e. taking three packets without a break, using the lowest acceptable fixed dose formulation (note that triphasic COCs cannot be used in this way). This means that the woman has only five such migraines a year instead of 13. Continuous use of COCs is another option, although breakthrough bleeding is more likely than with tricycling.

Migraine related to the pill-free interval is most notable in women taking contraceptives containing a relatively high proportion of progestogen. This can often be resolved by changing the formulation to a more oestrogen-dominant pill, for example changing Loestrin to Mercilon or Microgynon to Marvelon, provided there are no contraindications to the use of third-generation progestogens. Use of natural oestrogen supplements during the pill-free interval has anecdotal support but results of a double-blind placebo-controlled study are awaited.

Consideration should be given to stopping the pill, or changing to non-ethinyloestradiol contraception, if headaches are severe after tricycling or adding natural oestrogen, and certainly if there is concern about any change in symptoms.

Progestogen-only contraception

10

This includes the progestogen-only pill, injectable progestogens and the levonorgestrel intrauterine system. These methods have not been associated with an increased risk of thrombotic stroke and can be used by women with any type of migraine which contraindicates COC use. Women can be changed from COCs to progestogen-only contraception immediately, even during an attack.

No specific clinical trials have assessed the nature or frequency of migraine associated with progestogen-containing contraception although headache is a noted side-effect of these methods. This usually settles with continued use.

Emergency contraception

Use of combined ethinyloestradiol and progestogen emergency contraception (PC4) is not contraindicated for women with migraine, unless a woman with a history of migraine with aura is *currently* experiencing an attack of migraine (with or without aura), at the time of taking emergency contraception. In these cases progestogen-only emergency contraception, or an intrauterine device, may be more appropriate.

Migraine and pregnancy

Approximately 70% of migraineurs improve during pregnancy, particularly during the second and third trimester, although attacks often return with menstruation. The mechanism is often considered to be the rising levels of sex hormones. It is unlikely that the true mechanism is so simple as there are many physical, biochemical and emotional changes in pregnancy, which could account for improvement. These include altered glucose tolerance, reduced muscular tension and elevated pain threshold.

However, it is not uncommon for migraine to start *de novo* during pregnancy and women with pre-existing migraine may develop aura for the first time. The development of typical aura does not appear to be associated with sinister sequelae; neither does migraine pose any threat to the pregnancy.

Ideally, preparation for pregnancy should begin before conception as many drugs and other teratogens exert their greatest effects on the fetus in the first trimester, often before the woman knows she is pregnant. Prophylactic medication should be discontinued and strategies for the management of acute attacks discussed.

It is useful to extend advice to postpartum management. Although migraine does not typically return until menstruation recommences, the immediate postpartum period is a time of increased risk. A few women experience frequent attacks while breast-feeding.

Ideally, drugs should be avoided and attacks prevented and treated with non-drug methods. For acute treatment, paracetamol is the only drug that can safely be recommended throughout pregnancy and breast-feeding. For nausea, prochlorperazine is unlikely to cause harm throughout pregnancy and lactation. Metoclopramide and domperidone are probably safe during the second and third trimesters.

The use of prophylactics should be restricted but, if necessary, propranolol has the greatest weight of data assessing its safety during pregnancy and lactation.

All women using drug therapy, at any stage of pregnancy, should be counselled with regard to the relative risks and benefits of such treatment.

Differential diagnosis

Effective management is dependent on correct diagnosis of the headache. Cerebrovascular disorders may present with symptoms not dissimilar from migraine so a careful history and examination are

10

mandatory, particularly if symptoms change or the first attack starts during pregnancy. Non-migraine headaches can be associated with superimposed migraine attacks, in which case each headache should be treated separately.

Reassurance

Once the diagnosis of migraine has been confirmed, the first step in management is to reassure the patient that migraine does not pose any threat the baby. This is particularly important for women with classical migraine or whose attacks convert from common to classical during pregnancy as these symptoms can be frightening.

Non-drug treatments

Recognition of triggers with the aid of diary cards and subsequent avoidance is the obvious way to prevent attacks, without the need for medication. However, many symptoms of early pregnancy can aggravate migraine. Pregnancy sickness, particularly if severe, can reduce food and fluid intake resulting in low blood sugar and dehydration. Simple advice to eat small, frequent carbohydrate snacks and drink plenty of fluids may help both problems. Adequate rest is recommended to counter overtiredness, particularly in the first and last trimesters. Other preventative measures that can be safely tried include yoga, biofeedback techniques, massage and stress management.

Simple measures for managing acute attacks can be surprisingly effective: alternating hot and cold compresses applied to the site of pain; an ice-pack (a bag of frozen peas is effective, provided it is covered with a cloth to prevent frostbite) or heat pad on the back of the neck; lying in a quiet, darkened room.

Herbal remedies

Many people perceive herbal remedies to be safe because they are natural. However, medicinal herbs can be powerful drugs. Some are specifically used to induce abortion and others have been linked to miscarriage. For these reasons, herbal medicines should be avoided unless recommended by a qualified practitioner.

Medication in pregnancy and during lactation

As a general principle, avoid administering any drug during early pregnancy and, throughout pregnancy, only recommend drugs if the benefit clearly outweighs the possible risks to the fetus.

Few drugs have been tested for safety in pregnancy and during breast-feeding because of the obvious ethical limitations of undertaking clinical trials. Therefore, bear in mind that the manufacturers do not generally recommend the use of any drug in pregnancy because of insufficient data.

Women who have taken their usual migraine treatment will be concerned about the effects of these, and other drugs, on the pregnancy. Early pregnancy loss through natural causes is high but many women wrongly blame themselves if they miscarry. Although they can be reassured that it is rare for drugs commonly used in migraine to have detrimental effects on the fetus, future drug treatment should be limited.

Analgesics

Aspirin

Clinical and epidemiological data from large numbers of women who have taken analgesic doses of aspirin during pregnancy provide evidence of its safety in the first and second trimester of pregnancy. It should be used with caution near term as its effect on platelet function increases the risk of prolonged labour, postpartum haemorrhage and neonatal bleeding. In common with all prostaglandin synthetase inhibitors, aspirin may cause premature closure of the fetal ductus arteriosus. Aspirin is excreted in breast milk so breast-feeding mothers should avoid its use because of the theoretical risk of Reye's syndrome and impaired platelet function in susceptible infants, although occasional use by the mother is unlikely to cause adverse effects.

Paracetamol

Epidemiological evidence is sufficient to show that paracetamol can safely be given to pregnant and breast-feeding women, although its effects in these women has not been studied as extensively as those of aspirin. It is the mild analgesic of choice in pregnancy.

Codeine

Respiratory malformation in neonates may be associated with codeine exposure during pregnancy and codeine excreted in the breast milk can cause sedation and respiratory depression. However, occasional use at doses found in combined analgesics is unlikely to cause harm.

Non-steroidal anti-inflammatory drugs

There are insufficient data to support the use of most NSAIDs in pregnant and breast-feeding women. However, reproduction studies on white rabbits given ibuprofen have not shown any treatment-related abnormalities and the drug has been safely given during pregnancy at doses not exceeding 600 mg/day for the management of rheumatoid arthritis. Other effects are similar to those of aspirin. The concentration of ibuprofen in breast milk is very low and is therefore unlikely to affect the infant.

Antiemetics

Buclizine

This is an antihistamine combined with paracetamol and codeine in proprietary migraine treatments, available in many countries without prescription. Buclizine is not recommended in pregnancy as studies of high doses in rats have shown teratogenic effects including cleft palate. However, in clinical practice it has been in wide use for many years without apparent adverse effects. Minimal levels pass into breast milk so it can be taken during breast-feeding.

Cyclizine

This is also widely available without prescription alone or in combination with analgesics, for the treatment of migraine. It is a possible teratogen although this concern has not been substantiated in prospective controlled studies.

Domperidone

Variable embryotoxic effects have occurred in animal tests but a causal link with domperidone has not been confirmed. A study of 50 pregnant women treated over 20 days between the fourth and 12th week of pregnancy showed no adverse outcome. Minimal amounts are excreted into breast milk and domperidone is occasionally prescribed to improve postnatal lactation.

10

Metoclopramide

This has not shown any teratogenic effect in clinical experience or in animal studies. Only small amounts are found in breast milk and are unlikely to produce adverse effects.

Prochlorperazine

This has been widely used without ill effect and animal studies have not shown any teratogenic effect.

Vasoconstrictors

Ergotamine

This is contraindicated in pregnancy as animal studies have shown that its use is associated with increased perinatal mortality and developmental anomalies, including cleft palate and limb defects. This is thought to be due to ergotamine's potent vasoconstrictor action, impairing uteroplacental blood flow. It is also an abortifacient so should only be given to women using effective contraception. Ergotamine should not be taken during breast-feeding as it inhibits lactation.

Dihydroergotamine

This is not a known teratogen but with limited data available its use in pregnancy and during breast-feeding is not recommended.

Triptans

There is no evidence of teratogenicity in animal studies and there have been no reports of abnormalities in the babies delivered to the small numbers of women who have taken triptans during pregnancy. With such limited exposure, the use of triptans cannot be recommended during pregnancy and breast-feeding until more data are available, although the riazatriptan data sheet suggests that infant exposure can be minimized by avoiding breast-feeding for 24 h after treatment.

10

Prophylactics

Amitriptyline

This has been used for management of major depressive illness during pregnancy when the illness may affect the well being of the mother. For migraine it is probably best avoided and should not be used during the first and last trimesters. A few cases of limb deformity have been reported but this finding has not been confirmed by the results of national surveys. Tachycardia, irritability, muscle spasms and convulsions have occasionally been reported in the neonate. Amitriptyline and its active metabolite, nortriptyline, are detectable in breast milk but the effects on the neonate are unknown.

Methysergide

This has uterogenic properties. Its use is contraindicated in pregnancy and during breast-feeding and it should only be given to women using effective contraception.

10

Pizotifen

This has not been associated with any reported embryotoxic or adverse effects during pregnancy although the data are limited. Safety during breast-feeding is not established although concentrations of pizotifen measured in breast milk are not likely to adversely affect the infant.

Propranolol

Safety in pregnancy is not established but propranolol has been widely taken with no evidence of teratogenicity and is the only prophylactic that can be recommended. Even so, its use should be restricted to severe cases not responding to non-drug management. Propranolol has been associated with growth retardation, hypoglycaemia, hypocalcaemia, bradycardia and respiratory depression. Since most women are given propranolol in pregnancy for the treatment of hypertension or eclampsia, it is difficult to know if the underlying condition, or the treatment, is the cause of these effects. Propranolol is excreted into breast milk and may cause bradycardia and hypoglycaemia in the infant. Other β-blockers have similar effects but data are even more limited.

Valproate

This is highly teratogenic. Its use is contraindicated in pregnancy and it should only be given to women using effective contraception. First-trimester use is associated with neural tube defects and a characteristic pattern of facial defects. The concentration found in breast milk is very low so it can be used during lactation.

Prescribing for the pregnant woman

There is a difference between reassuring the pregnant woman that what she has taken is unlikely to have affected the pregnancy, and advising her what she should take. All women should be counselled that there is only minimal information about the safety of most drugs during pregnancy. Use of any drug is a balance of relative risks and benefits. For acute treatment, paracetamol is safe throughout pregnancy and lactation. Aspirin is also safe, but may cause bleeding problems if taken near term. Prochlorperazine has been used for pregnancy-related nausea for many years. Metoclopramide and domperidone are safe, but are probably best avoided during the first trimester. If frequent attacks occur during the first trimester, most women can be reassured that migraine improves during the second and third trimester. For continuing frequent attacks which warrant prophylaxis, propranolol has best evidence of safety during pregnancy and lactation.

References

1 MacGregor EA. Menstruation, sex hormones and headache. *Neurol Clin* 1997; 15: 125–41.
2 Somerville BW. Estrogen withdrawal migraine. *Neurology* 1975; 25: 239–50.
3 Guillebaud J. *Contraception Today.* London, Martin Dunitz, 1997.
4 Tzourio C, Tehindrazanarivelo A, Iglésias S *et al.* Case-control study of migraine and risk of ischaemic stroke in young women. *BMJ* 1995; 310: 830–3.
5 MacGregor EA, Guillebaud J. Recommendations for clinical practice: combined oral contraceptives, migraine and stroke. *Br J Fam Planning* 1998; 24: 53–60.

CHAPTER 11

Other Groups: Children, Men and the Elderly

Children and adolescents

Migraine is the most common cause of benign recurrent headache in children and is associated with a high burden of morbidity. Although it typically starts during the teens or early twenties, it can occur in very young children. Despite its high prevalence, migraine is frequently underdiagnosed. Few children are seen by their GP and even fewer receive either a diagnosis or advice on effective management strategies.

Headache and migraine prevalence (Table 11.1)

The most comprehensive study on migraine and headache prevalence was undertaken by Bille in Uppsala, Sweden, during 1955 [1]. He studied all schoolchildren aged between 7 and 15 years who attended one of the Uppsala primary or secondary schools. A questionnaire was given to these 9059 children to take home to their parents, the aim being to determine whether the children suffered headaches. From the 8993 replies Bille showed that the overall prevalence of headache was 59%. The preva-

11

Table 11.1 Epidemiology of migraine in children and adolescents.

Author	Age group	No. studied	Migraine prevalence (%)
Valqhuist [22]	10–12	1236	4.5
Bille [1]	7–15	8993	4
Sillanpää [23]	7	1927	1.9
Sillanpää & Piekkala [24]	14	3863	10.2
Mortimer et al. [25]	3–11	1083	3.7–4.9*
Abu-Arefeh & Russell [26]	5–15	1754	10.6–11.3*
Metsahonkala & Sillanpää [27]	8–9	3580	2.7–3.5*
Sillanpää & Anttila [4]	7	1433	5.7

*Figures vary according to criteria used.

lence of migraine in 7-year-olds was 1.4% with a mean age at onset of 4.8 years. By the ages of 7–9 years migraine prevalence was ≈2.5% in both boys and girls; by 15 migraine prevalence had increased to 5.3%. Before puberty there was no difference between the sexes in the incidence of migraine but after the age of 11 there was an increasing female predominance which became more marked in the 13–15 age group.

This female preponderance was also shown in a study of Aberdeen schoolchildren showing a prevalence of 10.6% in a group of 2165 children aged 5–15 [2]. Prevalence increased with age, with male preponderance in children under 12 and female preponderance thereafter. A different study suggests that the type of migraine is also gender specific; population survey data from the large Washington County study showed that it is migraine without aura which rises at the onset of menarche [3].

Studies from Finland highlight the concern that migraine and headache are increasing in prevalence. In 1974, of 1927 7-year-olds starting school, the prevalence of migraine was 1.9%. In a similar study of 1436 7-year-olds undertaken by the same primary author in the same school in 1992, 22 years later, migraine prevalence had increased to 5.7% [4]. The overall prevalence of headache had substantially increased being only 14.4% in 1974 compared with 51.5% by 1992. Although the exact reasons for this increasing prevalence is unknown, increased stresses and rushed snacks replacing proper meals are two noticeable problems of recent years.

Effect of migraine on time lost from school

Severe pain and associated symptoms, particularly vomiting which is often aggravated by movement, may mean children have to remain at home during attacks and are unable to participate in normal daily ac-

Table 11.2 Diagnostic criteria. Paediatric migraine without aura. Adapted from Winner P, Martinez W, Mate L, Bello L. Classification of pediatric migraine: proposed revision to the IHS criteria. *Headache* 1995; 35: 407–10.

Headache lasts 30 min to 48 h
Headache has at least two of the following:
  Bilateral (frontal/temporal) or unilateral location
  Pulsating quality
  Moderate to severe intensity
  Aggravation by routine physical activity
During headache, at least one of the following:
  Nausea and/or vomiting
  Photophobia and/or phonophobia

Table 11.3 Diagnostic criteria. Paediatric migraine with aura. Adapted from Winner P, Martinez W, Mate L, Bello L. Classification of pediatric migraine: proposed revision to the IHS criteria. *Headache* 1995; 35: 407–10.

At least three of the following:
One or more fully reversible aura symptoms indicating focal cortical and/or brainstem dysfunction
At least one aura symptom developing gradually over more than 4 min or, 2 or more symptoms occurring in succession
No aura lasting more than 60 min
Headache follows aura with a free interval of less than 60 min

tivities. If such attacks are frequent, migraine can have a significant detrimental effect on schooling. In one study children with migraine lost a mean of 7.8 days a year due to all illnesses compared with a mean of 3.7 days lost by controls [2]. Whether the problem with migraine stems from difficulties at school or vice versa needs consideration.

Clinical features of migraine in children

Missing the diagnosis of migraine can occur if adult migraine diagnostic criteria are used for children as there are important differences between childhood migraine and adult migraine (Tables 11.2 & 11.3).

11

The main differences from adult migraine are:
- attacks are shorter in children, sometimes lasting less than an hour;
- headache is typically bilateral, rather than unilateral;
- headache may be only a minor symptom gastrointestinal symptoms such as nausea and vomiting and, particularly, abdominal pain are much more prominent [5].

Making the diagnosis (Table 11.4)

Recurrent bouts of headache with nausea or vomiting, with complete

Table 11.4 Differential diagnosis: children.

Acute headache		Recurrent headache	
Common	Rare	Common	Rare
See Recurrent	Meningitis	Muscle contraction	Intracranial pathology
Sinusitis	Encephalitis	Migraine	
Dental	Intracranial	Emotional tension	
Traumatic (including	pathology	Medication misuse	
non-accidental injury			

freedom from symptoms between attacks, may be migraine. Some children may look pale and yawn a few hours before the headache starts; others are bursting with extra energy. Some children may experience an aura, typically visual, before the headache. Vomiting or sleep typically resolve the attack. Parents and carers are often surprised at how quickly children recover.

Children should be given the opportunity to describe symptoms for themselves. It is a common misconception that children are unable to describe migraine, as even those as young as 3 can give very accurate picture of a typical attack either verbally or pictorially. As in adults, there is no diagnostic test for migraine, so diagnosis depends entirely on the history and examination.

A headache diary can aid diagnosis of headache and clarify features of attacks that are not picked up by the history. It can be used to help children identify warning prodromal symptoms. It is particularly valuable in establishing the presence of additional headaches which can be the cause of treatment failure if not recognized and managed appropriately. This is covered in more detail in Chapter 8.

Is it something more serious?

Abnormal neurological signs are present in ≈95% of tumour patients presenting with new onset of headache in the previous 2–4 months. Increased frequency or severity of headache and occurrence on waking, particularly if associated with seizures, are also indicate a possible tumour.

When called out to a child with headache consider:
• is the history of this headache consistent with similar past episodes of a benign cause such as migraine (recurrent episodic symptoms with the child completely well between attacks)—in which case, treat as migraine, with early review.
• are there any unusual features of concern (persistent vomiting, fever, meningism, altered consciousness, seizure, abnormal neurological findings)—refer to hospital immediately providing any immediate supportive treatment such as parenteral penicillin if menigococcal meningitis is suspected.

When to refer for investigation

It is wise to have a low threshold for referral for investigation of recent headaches, i.e. headaches starting within the last 6 months, or headache in a child under the age of 6.

Other indications for further investigation are:
- alteration in character of headache;
- an unaccountable increase in frequency, severity and duration of attacks;
- recent school failure;
- personality changes;
- failure to grow/attain normal developmental goals;
- fits with headache;
- abnormal neurological symptoms during or after headache;
- new neurological symptoms;
- abnormality on neurological examination.

Long-standing headaches or headaches in a child over the age of seven, provided the clinical examination is normal, can be observed.

Management of migraine

Migraine in children is essentially managed in the same way as migraine in adults.

One major hurdle to effective management is that recurrent episodic headache in children is frequently not recognized as migraine either by parents or by doctors. This is more probable for migraine without aura (common migraine) which is often just seen as a 'sick' headache or 'bilious attack'. Migraine with aura (classical migraine) is much easier to identify with its dramatic heralding 'aura'. Even when parents have recognized the condition, they often still do not consult a doctor, in the mistaken belief that little can be done about migraine. Another concern of parents is that an ill child may play on their illness and use it to avoid going to school [6].

Management of migraine is often inadequate with one study showing that many children do not use any medication during attacks. This is despite the fact that the majority have to go to bed while many experience attacks severe enough to make them cry with the pain [6]. But drug treatments are only one aspect of management. Children, as much as parents, can be quite concerned about their headaches and have clear views about management.

The main concerns that need addressing are:
- the cause of the headaches;
- what will make the headaches better;
- reassurance that they do not have a brain tumour.

11

The cause

Just as in adults, migraine is triggered by a combination of events, not just a single event. Children themselves are often aware of relevant triggers, typically lack of sleep, exercise, delayed or missed meals, and worries about home or school. Be on the alert for parental conflicts or bullying. These are important triggers in children which are easily overlooked. Sensitive counselling is necessary in these situations.

Identifying more typical triggers requires motivation but is not complicated. Children can be asked to keep a daily trigger diary recording any event that is different from their normal routine, or which they feel may be relevant. This can include missed meals, sports activities, stressful lessons, late-night study, emotional upsets, etc. A record of migraine attacks and other headaches should be kept separate from this. After a few months, the parents and children can look through the diaries, noting patterns of any build of triggers, or specific triggers, preceding attacks. Having identified possible culprits, their relevance can be assessed by avoiding them, one at a time, over subsequent months. Clearly, it is impossible to avoid all potential triggers but it is unnecessary to do so; by minimizing the effects of just one or two it may be possible to remain below the attack threshold. Children can also learn which situations are more likely to provoke attacks enabling them to treat attacks early.

Inadequate nutrition is probably the major trigger in this age group, particularly during the adolescent growth spurt. It is not uncommon for children to rush off to school after an inadequate breakfast, taking a packed lunch that they do not eat because they would rather play games in the lunch hour. It is not surprising that many children develop a headache by late afternoon. Parents should make an effort to provide their children with a proper breakfast so that, even if they do miss lunch, at least they have been set up for the day.

Food allergy in children is contentious. Missed meals make a child more likely to crave sweets or chocolate, and sweet cravings are a common prodromal symptom of migraine. It is not surprising therefore that chocolate has been wrongly blamed as a migraine trigger. A few susceptible children have established a definite and reproducible temporal relationship between the consumption of certain foods and the onset of migraine, but such foods are usually identified by recording a food diary. In some cases, a trial of an oligoantigenic diet may be valuable. For the majority, it is unnecessary to restrict food and much more important to ensure that children have a sensible and regular diet.

11

Sport can also trigger attacks, probably by effects on blood sugar. Glucose tablets before and during sport can help in addition to supplementing meals with mid-morning and mid-afternoon snacks.

Making the headache better

Acute treatment

Simple non-drug treatments such as resting in a quiet, darkened room, using a hot or cold pack to ease the pain, and gentle massage, may be sufficient to control mild symptoms. Most children want to lie down during an attack and they should be encouraged to sleep as this can hasten recovery.

Drug treatment should be kept simple. If taken early in an attack, over-the-counter analgesia may be all that is necessary. Syrups should be given where possible. Soluble or effervescent analgesics can be dissolved in a sweet fizzy drink to make them more palatable and more effective. Treatment should be taken in adequate doses as early in an attack as possible since gastric stasis can delay absorption of drugs, reducing efficacy.

It is advisable to inform the child's school about the problem. It is helpful to provide staff with specific written instructions for management, stressing the need for early treatment. Schools have different rules regarding treatment. In some schools, teachers and/or nurses may agree to administer some medication. In other cases, the school will telephone the carer to collect the child.

More detail relating to drug therapy for migraine can be found in Chapter 8.

Paracetamol (Table 11.5) is probably the drug of choice as it can be given as a syrup to even very young children. It is also available as a suppository. Ibuprofen and other non-steroidal anti-inflammatory drugs (NSAIDs) are alternatives. Aspirin is not recommended for children under 12 in the UK. Migraleve is an over-the-counter tablet for children

Table 11.5 Over-the-counter oral analgesics.

Analgesic	Age (years)	Dose (mg)	Max. dose (24 h)
Paracetamol	1–5	120–250 every 4–6 h	4 doses
	6–12	250–500 every 4–6 h	
Ibuprofen	1–2	50 every 4–6 h	20 mg/kg in
	3–7	100 every 4–6 h	divided doses
	8–12	200 every 4–6 h	

Table 11.6 Pro-kinetic antiemetics.

Antiemetic	Weight (kg)	Dose (mg)
Domperidone (oral)		0.2–0.4 mg/kg every 4–8 h
Domperidone (rectal)	10–15	15 every 12 h
	15.5–25	30 every 12 h
	25.5–35	30 every 8 h
	35.5–45	30 every 6 h
Metoclopramide (oral)	10–14	1 every 8–12 h
	15–19	2 every 8–12 h
	20–29	2.5 every 8 h
	≥ 30	5 every 8 h

over age 10, combining paracetamol, codeine and buclizine, which can help nausea. It can also be prescribed to younger children. If necessary, analgesics can be combined with a pro-kinetic antiemetic such as domperidone or metoclopramide to promote normal gastric motility as well as controlling nausea (Table 11.6). Although not licensed for migraine, domperidone can be used in children over the age of 2. Metoclopramide can help to promote sleep but should be used very cautiously in children because of the increased risk of dystonic reactions. Drugs containing opiates or opiate derivatives should be avoided as these can aggravate nausea and vomiting.

If vomiting prohibits oral treatment, suppositories of paracetamol and domperidone can be used. NSAID suppositories are also helpful in older children (Table 11.7).

More specific migraine drugs, such as ergotamine or the triptans, are not recommended for use in children as there is insufficient data on safety in this age group. There is some evidence that these drugs may be less effective in children than in adults [7].

Prophylaxis (Table 11.8)

Non-drug treatments are of primary importance. Identification and

Table 11.7 Prescription NSAIDs.

Analgesic	Age	Dose (mg/kg)
Diclofenac	1–12	1–3 in 2 divided doses
Naproxen	Only over 5 years	10 in 2 divided doses

Table 11.8 Prophylactic drugs.

Drug	Starting dose (mg)	Max. daily dose (mg)
Cyproheptadine*	age 2–6 years: 2 *nocte*	4
	age 7–14 years: 4 *nocte*	8
Pizotifen	0.5 *nocte*	1.5
Propranolol	10 once or twice daily	60

*Not licensed for use in children in the UK.

management of trigger factors are the mainstay of treatment. Children also respond well to biofeedback and relaxation techniques which should be considered before instigating drug therapy.

It is rarely necessary to give prophylactic medication as the clinical course of primary headache is such that the headaches tend to improve spontaneously. Therefore drug therapy should never be given unless the headaches are really disabling. For a minority, a short course of prophylactic drugs may be indicated when there is concern that attacks are interfering with normal school work—often around exam time. The child should try them out before the critical time to ensure that the drug can be tolerated and side-effects do not compromise performance. The most commonly prescribed prophylactics for children are propranolol and pizotifen, with pizotifen being the drug of choice [5]. Cyproheptadine may also be used.

Reassurance

It is very important to reassure the child and parents that there is nothing seriously wrong. As with adults, many parents fear that if their child has headaches they may be due to a serious condition such as a brain tumour. A typical history of migraine and normal neurological examination provide evidence of the benign nature of the headache and therefore, in most cases, further investigation is not indicated.

When treatment fails

If children are experiencing frequent attacks of migraine or headache, particularly if these are not responding to simple management strategies, reconsider the diagnosis and consider further investigation.

Depression is often not recognized in children and should be considered in any child who has lost weight, become withdrawn, and has disrupted sleep, in whom no organic cause for the symptoms can be found. Bullying at school, emotional problems, etc. should also be sought and managed appropriately.

Overuse of acute medication should be considered. Even paracetamol alone may be responsible [8]. Acute treatment should not be used regularly on more than 2–3 days a week for more than 3 months. This is easily identified by asking the child or parents to keep a daily record of headache and treatments taken. Initial management is withdrawal of all analgesic drugs with explanation to the child and to the parents. This alone is often associated with marked improvement. Refractory cases may require psychiatric referral.

Recurrent abdominal pain and migraine

The term 'abdominal migraine' is considered to describe attacks of periodic abdominal pain which may occur with or without cranial symptoms [9]. With advancing age, abdominal symptoms associated with episodic headache accompanied by photophobia, nausea and vomiting, become less prominent with loss of abdominal pain in adulthood. Such cases should be treated as migraine.

Whether recurrent abdominal pain without associated typical migraine symptoms reflects a true association with migraine is uncertain. It is common in children: 8.4% in a study of 1104 children registered with a general practice [6] and occurs in many other medical conditions, including irritable bowel or even coeliac disease, which may be more relevant.

Therefore, full investigation should be made to exclude other causes first. 'Recurrent abdominal pain of childhood' is probably a more accurate term and should be reserved for recurrent, stereotyped attacks of abdominal pain lasting for a few hours at the most, with no symptoms between attacks. In practice, most cases of otherwise unexplained recurrent abdominal pain have an underlying psychosomatic basis and would benefit from more appropriate treatment [10].

Motion sickness and migraine

Motion sickness is often linked to migraine. One study suggested that motion sickness was an associated feature in 45% of children with migraine, a figure which was seven times higher than control groups [11]. However, since travel is a trigger for migraine, the true association is uncertain.

154

Prognosis of migraine

Migraine is a condition with marked fluctuations in frequency and severity of attacks over time. Bille has followed his cohort of 73 schoolchildren with severe attacks of migraine, initially aged between 7 and 13, over 40 years [12]. His results showed that a migrainous child has a 60% chance of remission in adolescence. Freedom from attacks may last for several years but recurrence is common; by the age of 50 more than half of the group still had migraine. Adult attacks tended to be less frequent and less severe than in childhood.

The type of migraine can also change with time, many people losing the aura and some developing aura without an ensuing headache.

Summary

Simple management strategies learned young are important as they can be used and developed to control migraine effectively in later life. Education is the key to effective management. In the majority of cases, doctors need do little more than establish the diagnosis, reassure the child and parents, in addition to providing information about how to identify potential triggers and advice on effective drug therapy. If there is any uncertainty about the diagnosis or if the attacks do not respond to simple management strategies, consider referral to a paediatrician, preferably with an interest in headache.

11

Case study

Ben is 14 and has had common migraine since he was 8. Attacks used to be infrequent but for the last couple of months he has been having attacks most weeks, often starting late afternoon when he gets in from school. He develops a left or right-sided headache associated with nausea and photophobia. His mother says he looks very pale and has to go to bed. A couple of hours in to the attack, he vomits and then feels much better. He can then take a couple of paracetamol and goes to sleep. By the next morning, he is fine. His mother is concerned that these attacks are affecting his schoolwork, as he is not completing his homework. The doctor asks if Ben has needed new shoes or outgrown his clothes recently. His mother replies that he has been growing rapidly over the last few months and is eating her out of house and home. The doctor explains that growth spurts are a common time for migraine to worsen. The doctor asks Ben what he eats for lunch and which sports he enjoys. Ben replies, trying not to look at his mother, that he takes a packed lunch but has little time to eat it as he has football practice during the lunch hour. He often has further sports after school. The doctor points out that the body needs fuel in order to function ('You couldn't try to drive a car without petrol'). The doctor also recommends that Ben tries to eat more sensibly and keeps a record of attacks over the next few weeks. Ben and his mother return to report that his simple advice has been very effective, although it took a couple of weeks before they noticed any improvement. Ben also comments that he has much more energy after school.

Comment

Keep treatment simple in children and be cautious about prescribing medication, particularly for prophylaxis. Identification and management of relevant trigger factors should be the first consideration.

Men

Much of the information regarding diagnosis and management of migraine in men is covered in other sections. However, there are a few differences of note.

Fewer men then women with migraine consult a doctor [13]. This is perhaps because attacks are milder in men [14]. Attacks often occur at weekends so they are less likely to disrupt work.

Overall, there is a lower prevalence of migraine in males compared to females, the lifetime prevalence being 8%. Migraine in males more often starts before the age of 10 and attacks are more likely to be with aura compared with females.

The main time of difficulty with migraine for boys is during the growth spurt at puberty. Adequate regular nutrition is often all that is necessary. Sport is also a common trigger in this group, particularly sustained physical exercise such as football or cross-country running. The simplest strategy for prevention is to maintain glucose levels with glucose sweets, drink fluids to avoid dehydration, and take exercise gradually and progressively where possible. If symptoms are progressive, other possible causes to exclude are phaeochromocytoma, and intracranial lesions or stenosis of the carotid arteries. Minor blows to the head during sport, such as heading a football or a hit on the face in a rugby tackle, can trigger an instantaneous migraine aura, not always followed by headache [15]. Such attacks have been shown to be benign.

Headache associated with sexual activity affects men more than women, more common in those who have migraine or hypertension

[16]. There is also a link with exercise headache. The commonest symptom is a dull occipital headache, probably related to excessive muscular contraction of the head and neck. This can be prevented by deliberate relaxation of the muscles, but may require pre-emptive treatment with an anti-inflammatory drug such as naproxen or propranolol [17]. Of more concern are headaches of explosive onset, also known as 'thunderclap headache', which mimic subarachnoid haemorrhage. Computed tomography scanning and cerebrospinal fluid examination are advised.

Work and the working environment can affect migraine in men. Work can also be affected by migraine as the condition is a significant cause of reduced productivity and sick leave. Time pressures and other stresses at work may be significant triggers that are further affected by frequent migraine. These problems need to be considered by occupational health physicians as well as by primary care physicians. This is discussed in more detail in Chapter 15.

Cluster headache is a specific type of headache that is more prevalent in men, although it is rare. This is discussed in Chapter 14.

Headache may be a presenting complaint of underlying psychosocial problems such as alcoholism, drug abuse, depression and marital conflicts. This is more typically tension-type headache than migraine, and management is directed to the underlying problem. The diagnosis of tension-type headache is also discussed in Chapter 14.

Although consultation time is often short, it is worthwhile questioning men about headache even when they are consulting for other reasons. Recognition of the true nature of any frequent headaches coupled with simple advice on management strategies can reduce morbidity from migraine.

The elderly

It is very unusual for migraine to start *de novo* in later life and it typically improves in both frequency and severity in both sexes after the age of 55. The mechanism for this may relate to progressive impairment of cerebral vasodilator capacitance with advancing age [18]. The character of attacks may change with loss of headache in attacks of migraine with aura. Such attacks my be confused with transient ischaemic attacks (TIAs) if a past history of migraine with similar aura symptoms has not been elicited.

Non-migraine headaches remain common and advancing age is associated with an increasing likelihood that headache may be a symptom of a more serious problem. If the history is typical of migraine and there are no relevant findings on examination, further investigation is rarely helpful to the diagnosis [19]. However, whenever patients report a change from their typical pattern of headache or develop unusual symptoms, a careful history and examination can elicit or rule out headaches related to underlying disease. Fundoscopic examination is mandatory at first presentation with headache and is worth repeating.

Headache as a side-effect of other treatment

An often unrecognized cause of headache in elderly people is side-effects of medication taken for chronic disorders. This is particularly the case for vasodilator drugs used for the treatment of ischaemic heart disease such as nifedipine, glyceryl trinitrate and isosorbide dinitrate. There is long list of other drugs reputed to induce headache [20]. Some drugs used for hypertension can worsen headache but others, such as β-blockers, can treat both. It is helpful to evaluate all drugs taken, reducing the dose and changing or stopping drugs where possible. Overuse of acute headache treatments is associated with frequent headache. This is discussed in Chapter 14.

Headache as a symptom of underlying disease

Disorders of the cervical spine

Both headache and migraine can be associated with cervical spondylosis. Pain can be referred to the orbital region from disorders affecting the upper three cervical roots such as rheumatoid arthritis or trauma. Occipital headache can arise from muscle contraction associated with osteoarthritis of the upper cervical zygapophyseal joints. Treatment is necessarily conservative with anti-inflammatory agents and occasionally with immobilization. Manipulation, although popular, is potentially risky for this age group as it can result in dissection of the cerebral arteries with brainstem infarction. Acupuncture, or even local anaesthetic agents or steroids injected into the tender points can be helpful.

Dental problems

Poor dentition and ill-fitting dentures are often overlooked as a cause of facial pain that may mimic myalgic pain and migraine. Referral to a dentist is indicated if a dental cause is suspected. Temporomandibular joint disease resulting in tension in the muscles of mastication can trigger temporal pain. On examination, pressure on the temporomandibular joint (by pressing anteriorly with a finger in the external auditory canal) replicates the pain, particularly as the patient is asked to slowly open and close the jaw. Simple exercises to relax the temporal and masseter muscles can ease the pain and amitriptyline is also helpful. Underlying dental problems warrant referral to a dentist, otherwise referral to an orthodontic surgeon may be indicated to adjust the bite.

Depression

Depression is common in the elderly. Headache is associated with depression and may arise from lack of sleep and poor nutrition in addition to a reduced pain threshold and biochemical changes. Management includes social and psychological support. The reader is referred to other texts for specific management of depression in the elderly [21]. Antidepressives, although often prescribed, should be used with caution given the greater likelihood of adverse events in the elderly and the presence of comorbid conditions that may restrict their use.

Hypertension

Although many believe headache to be a common sign of hypertension, the blood pressure has to be very high with a diastolic greater than 130 mmHg before symptoms arise. A dull occipital headache is present on waking and gradually improves after rising. Sudden changes in blood pressure, such as those associated with a hypertensive crisis from monoamine oxidase inhibitors used for depression, or from phaeochromocytoma, give rise to pounding intermittent headache.

Temporal arteritis

Temporal arteritis rarely occurs under the age of 55. The prevalence during the fifties is around 6.8 per 100 000 and increases with age to affect 73 per 100 000 80-year-olds. The pain is unilateral and may be so intense that the patient cannot rest that side of the head on a pillow. Chewing may be painful and a history of weight loss or muscle pain suggests associated polymyalgia rheumatica. Fever, anorexia and fatigue may also occur. The temporal artery on the affected side is often prominent and tender but this is an unreliable sign. The optic discs may appear pale and swollen. An elevated erythrocyte sedimentation rate (ESR) greater than 50 mm/h is usually considered sufficient for a diagnosis but may be elevated in the elderly for other reasons. A biopsy is confirmatory. Symptoms respond to prednisolone within a few days. Because of the risk of blindness, high doses of prednisolone, initially

11

60–100 mg daily, should be started immediately in a patient with typical features, even before the biopsy. The dose should be reduced as the ESR falls.

Carbon monoxide poisoning

During the winter elderly people often use gas heaters, which may be faulty, without adequate ventilation. This can give rise to carbon monoxide poisoning. Symptoms include throbbing headache, fatigue, dizziness and nausea. Since the diagnosis is frequently missed, it is worth asking patients with non-specific headache about their heating! When on visits, GPs can spot gas fires which may be burning inefficiently and emitting carbon monoxide. The fire burns with a yellow flame instead of a blue one and deposits soot on the ceramic plate behind it. If suspected, the environmental health department should be contacted to inspect the property.

Trigeminal neuralgia

Trigeminal neuralgia typically starts in the elderly affecting slightly more women than men. The pain is restricted to the distribution of the trigeminal nerve, usually the second or third division. The pain is described as sudden spasms of severe shooting pain lasting only seconds— often described as like an electric shock. This occurs repeatedly in daily paroxysms for several weeks or months. Patients have often identified triggers such as chewing, cleaning the teeth, shaving and even cold wind on the face. Examination of cranial nerve function is normal. Carbamazepine is the drug of choice. Elderly patients should start with 100 mg/day in three to four divided doses (necessary because of the short half-life of the drug). This should be increased until symptomatic control is reached to a maximum of 400 mg three times daily, or until side-effects of giddiness or drowsiness limit higher doses. Treatment failure is usually due to an inadequate dose. Leucopenia nearly always occurs but is rarely of clinical significance. If carbamazepine is ineffective, phenytoin or baclofen may be tried. Around 20% continue to have intractable pain which may require referral for surgical treatment.

Stroke

Atherothrombotic disease affecting the carotid or vertebral arteries can trigger TIA or ischaemic stroke associated with headache. Stroke is discussed in more detail in Chapter 13.

Table 11.9 Coexisting disease and migraine treatment.

Coexistent disease	Contraindicated therapy
Uncontrolled hypertension/ atherosclerosis	Ergotamine and ergot derivatives Triptans
Asthma Obstructive airways disease Diabetes Heart failure	β-blockers
Cardiac arrhythmias Myocardial infarction Glaucoma	Tricyclic antidepressives
Gastrointestinal ulceration Bleeding	NSAIDs

Space-occupying lesions

Headache is rarely the only presenting symptom of intracranial tumour. This is discussed in more detail in Chapter 13.

Management of migraine in the elderly (Table 11.9)

Management is aimed at treatment of the underlying cause. Drug therapy should be kept to a minimum, where possible, particularly since many coexistent illnesses can restrict the use of certain migraine treatments. Elderly people do not tolerate drugs as well as other age groups, particularly if they also have impaired liver or kidney function, so minimal doses should be used. Drugs containing opiates should be avoided as these can cause confusion and sedation as well as aggravating constipation. Otherwise general management strategies for each specific headache are indicated.

Case study

Mr J. is 72. He is a widower and lives alone. He has not had problems with headaches before but over the last few months he has had headaches most days. They start in the back of his neck, on the left, and end up over his eye. They are worse in the morning and often improve over the course of the day. He has no other associated symptoms. He does not like taking painkillers, although they do work. On examination, affect was normal and he did not appear depressed. Physical and neurological examination was normal with the exception of tense, tender neck and shoulder muscles, particularly on the left. Neck movements were restricted. The doctor diagnosed muscle contraction headache and referred Mr J. for physiotherapy. The physiotherapist suggested that Mr J. should replace his mattress, which was over 20 years old, and should not prop his head up with too many pillows. Mr J. said that he had to have several pillows to stop the acid from his stomach. The physiotherapist suggested that he discuss these symptoms with his doctor. In the meantime, he could ask his son to raise the head of the bed with blocks. This would have a similar effect to using several pillows. Mr J. is taught gentle stretching exercises. After a few months of treatment, the headaches are under control.

Comment

Deterioration of the cervical spine with advancing age can result in muscular pain which, in turn, triggers headache. In a patient of this age, a careful history and examination are necessary to exclude other causes of headache. Once a physical cause is considered, physical management is indicated. Although drugs such as anti-inflammatories may have some short-term benefit, they are treating symptoms and not the cause. Further, side-effects are more common in the elderly.

11

References

1 Bille B. Migraine in school children. *Acta Paediatr Scand* 1962; 51 (Suppl. 136): 1–151.
2 Abu-Arefeh I, Russell G. Prevalence of headache and migraine in schoolchildren. *BMJ* 1994; 309: 765–9.
3 Stewart WF, Linet MS, Celentano DD *et al.* Age- and sex-specific rates of migraine with and without aura. *Am J Epidemiol* 1991; 134: 1111–20.
4 Sillanpää M, Anttila P. Increasing prevalence of headache in 7-year-old schoolchildren. *Headache* 1996; 36: 466–70.
5 Symon DNK, Russell G. The general paediatrician's view of migraine—a review of 250 cases. In: *Headache in Children and Adolescents.* Lanzi G, Balottin U, Cernibori A, eds. Amsterdam, Elsevier Science Publishers, 1989: 61–6.
6 Mortimer MJ, Kay J, Jaron A. Clinical epidemiology of childhood abdominal migraine in an urban general practice. *Dev Med Child Neurol* 1993; 35: 243–8.
7 Hämäläinen ML, Hoppu K, Santavuori P. Sumatriptan for migraine attacks in children: a randomized placebo-controlled study. Do children with migraine respond to oral sumatriptan differently from adults. *Neurology* 1997; 48: 1100–3.
8 Symon DNK. Twelve cases of analgesic headache. *Arch Dis Child* 1998; 78: 555–6.
9 Symon DNK, Russell G. Abdominal migraine: a childhood syndrome defined. *Cephalalgia* 1986; 6: 223–8.

10 Hotopf M, Carr S, Mayou R, Wadsworth M, Wessely S. Why do children have chronic abdominal pain, and what happens to them when they grow up? Population based cohort study. *BMJ* 1998: 316; 1196–200.

11 Barabas G, Matthews WS, Ferrari M. Childhood migraine and motion sickness. *Paediatrics* 1983; 72: 188–90.

12 Bille BA. 40-year follow-up of school children with migraine. *Cephalalgia* 1997; 17: 488–91.

13 Rasmussen BK. Epidemiology of headache. *Cephalalgia* 1995; 15: 45–68.

14 Alvarez WC. Some important features of migraine. *Headache* 1961; 1: 20–3.

15 Bennett DR, Fuenning SI, Sullivan G, Weber J. Migraine precipitated by head trauma in athletes. *Am J Sports Med* 1980; 8: 202–5.

16 Dexter SL. study of coital related headaches in 32 patients. *Cephalalgia* 1985; 5: 299–300.

17 Porter M, Jankovic J. Benign coital cephalgia. Differential diagnosis and treatment. *Arch Neurol* 1981; 38: 710–2.

18 Meyer JS, Terayama Y, Konno S *et al.* Age-related cerebrovascular disease alters the symptomatic course of migraine. *Cephalalgia* 1998; 18: 202–8.

19 Cull RE. Investigation of late-onset migraine. *Scot Med J* 1995; 40: 50–2.

20 Lane RJ, Routledge PA. Drug-induced neurological disorders. *Drugs* 1983; 26: 124–47.

21 Lovestone S, Howard R. *Depression in Elderly People*. London, Martin Dunitz, 1997.

22 Vahlquist B. Migraine in children. *Int Arch Allergy* 1955; 7: 348–55.

23 Sillanpää M. Prevalence of migraine and other headache in children starting school. *Headache* 1976; 15: 288–90.

24 Sillanpää M, Piekkala P. Prevalence of migraine and other headaches in early puberty. *Scand J Prim Health Care* 1984; 2: 27–32.

25 Mortimer MJ, Kay J, Jaron A. Epidemiology of headache and childhood migraine in an urban general practice using Ad Hoc, Vahlquist and IHS criteria. *Dev Med Child Neurol* 1992; 34: 1095–101.

26 Abu-Arefeh I, Russell G. Prevalence of headache and migraine in school-children. *BMJ* 1994; 309: 765–9.

27 Metsahonkala L, Sillanpää M. Migraine in children—an evaluation of the IHS criteria. *Cephalalgia* 1994; 14: 285–90.

11

CHAPTER 12

Comorbid Conditions

Most patients have more than one disease. When an individual has two conditions which have a greater than coincidental association, the term comorbidity is used. Migraine is comorbid with a number of neurological and psychiatric conditions including anxiety, depression, asthma, epilepsy and stroke.

The coexistence of different diseases has important implications for diagnosis and management. For example, patients presenting with headache may be depressed. But does one condition cause the other, in which case, which do you treat first? Or do you try to treat both problems with one drug? Then there is the problem of which drug? Migraine prophylaxis with a β-blocker could aggravate depression whereas an antidepressant may be effective for both ailments. Similarly, in a patient with migraine and epilepsy, an antidepressant could lower the threshold to epileptic fits but sodium valproate would be an effective option.

The aim of this chapter is to highlight the main disorders that should be considered in any patient presenting with migraine. Simple questions can raise suspicion of comorbid conditions. For example, loss of appetite or early morning wakening suggest depression, prompting more specific enquiry. Management strategies can then be developed to maximize therapy with the minimum number of drugs. This reduces the likelihood of side-effects and drug interactions, in addition to reducing medication costs.

Depression and anxiety

Antidepressant drugs are often used in the management of chronic pain conditions, including headache. Studies suggest that they are effective in migraine regardless of whether or not depression is present [1]. Certainly, evidence exists that antidepressant agents have direct effects on pain, independent of their antidepressant actions.

The link between migraine and depression is complex. Prodromal symptoms occurring hours or days before the onset of headache often include mood changes, more often depression than elation. However, studies using standardized diagnostic criteria for depression, the DSM-

12

IV, consistently confirm a link between migraine and both unipolar depression and bipolar disorders. A similar link has been shown between migraine and anxiety. The association is not surprising given that these conditions are the result of disturbances in the same neurochemical system.

Implications for treatment

The only antidepressant with established efficacy in migraine is the tricyclic drug amitriptyline. The effective prophylactic dose varies considerably between subjects but low doses are generally used, starting at 10 mg taken at night. If this dose is ineffective, it is increased by 10 mg every 2 weeks to a usual daily dose between 20 and 150 mg. This should be continued for a 4–6-month course. Doses for migraine prophylaxis are lower than those used for the treatment of depression so if depression is evident or suspected, higher doses should be considered. Treatment may need to be continued for a year or longer.

Phenelzine, a monoamine oxidase inhibitor, is occasionally used in migraine but evidence of efficacy is limited and side-effects are common. More importantly, this class of drugs may potentiate the actions of foods containing tyramine and several drugs, possibly with a fatal outcome. Several of the interacting drugs are also used in migraine: tricyclic antidepressants, selective serotonin re-uptake inhibitors (SSRIs) and other 5-hydroxytryptamine (5HT) re-uptake inhibitors, and the acute drugs sumatriptan and zolmitriptan. Considering these problems, there is very little reason to recommend the use of phenelzine in migraine.

The antiepileptic sodium valproate is also used in the management of mood disorders and panic disorders. This may account for some of its efficacy in migraine prophylaxis.

Epilepsy

There have been conflicting data to support any relationship between epilepsy and migraine other than random coincidence. A recent meta-analysis of studies of the prevalence of epilepsy in people with migraine reported a median prevalence of 5.9%—far greater than the 1-year prevalence of 0.5% in the general population.

The reasons for this association are unclear. It has been proposed that an altered brain state may increase the risk of both migraine and epilepsy. Genetic or environmental risk factors may then increase neuronal excitability or reduce the threshold to attacks of both conditions. Certainly, many trigger factors are common to both migraine and

12

epilepsy, for example missed meals, alcohol, hormonal fluctuations and stress. A minority of patients report seizures during or immediately after migraine.

A structural lesion, such as an arteriovenous malformation (AVM) may precipitate migraine with aura, occasionally complicated by seizures. AVMs are congenital lesions which usually remain silent until mid-life at which time the patient can develop headaches, seizures and haemorrhages. Symptoms are unilateral, corresponding to the site of the AVM. This is unlike typical migraine, which is frequently associated with side-shift.

The diagnosis of epilepsy is usually obvious if tonic–clonic seizures have been witnessed or if there has been associated incontinence or tongue biting. Sometimes seizures may appear to mimic the symptoms of migraine. For example, benign occipital epilepsy can commence with visual symptoms although these are later followed by more obvious seizure manifestations such as hemiclonic movements. Postictal headache, nausea, vomiting and vertigo may follow. Temporal lobe epilepsy can be misdiagnosed as migraine with typical symptoms of *déjà vu* followed by a postictal headache. A careful history is necessary to distinguish the two conditions. The aura of epilepsy often includes a sensation of strange smell, or taste, auditory or visual hallucinations—not common to migraine. If the distinction between migraine and epilepsy is difficult, electroencephalogram (EEG) should be considered.

12

Case study

Julie was diagnosed with migraine at the age of 12. Treatment for migraine was unsuccessful and she was referred for psychotherapy. With symptoms continuing, the diagnosis was eventually reassessed when she was 22. Attacks commenced with an aura of visual and auditory (musical) hallucinations, and a dreamy state, sometimes accompanied by nausea and vertigo. This was followed by right-sided headache with nausea and vomiting lasting several hours. She was free from symptoms between attacks. Neurological examination was normal. The doctor recognized that hallucinations are not typical of migraine and referred her for further investigations. Her EEG recordings displayed primary epileptogenic areas in the right temporal and limbic lobes. The headache was synchronous with status discharges on EEG recordings.

Implications for treatment

Although the association is uncommon, patients with atypical migraine symptoms should be carefully assessed and may need referral to a specialist in order to exclude epilepsy. Patients at increased risk for both conditions include those with unusual or prolonged aura, particularly if symptoms include hallucinations, alterations of consciousness or positive motor symptoms. Headache without other neurological features is unlikely to be epilepsy.

If migraine and epilepsy coexist, treatment needs careful consideration. Migraine prophylactic agents such as the tricyclic antidepressants and the SSRIs can lower seizure threshold, provoking fits. Sodium valproate could be considered for the management of both conditions [2]. Counselling about precipitating factors—many of which are the same for both migraine and epilepsy—can also improve control.

Allergy and asthma

Several studies have identified a strong and consistent association between recognized allergic conditions and migraine, in both children and adults [3]. These studies have found a higher than expected prevalence of asthma.

Implications for treatment

An awareness of this association is important when considering drug therapy for migraine. Certain drugs, such as aspirin or β-blockers can provoke asthma and should be avoided if there is any reason to suspect such a reaction. Lifestyle management with identification and avoidance or treatments of particular stresses or other triggers for asthma and allergy will also help migraine. Suspected food allergy should be carefully managed to avoid malnutrition from food aversion. Food intolerance is more likely, although both are less common triggers for migraine than is often believed.

Stroke

The relationship between migraine and stroke is complicated by diagnostic confusion, particularly in patients with aura. The limited studies that have assessed the link are open to criticism related to selection of cases, definition of migraine and the problem of diagnosis. Controlled studies of patients with ischaemic stroke report a significantly increased risk of migraine. This association is greatest in women under age 45, particularly those with a history of migraine with aura. Studies suggest the absolute risk attributable to all types of migraine to be in

12

the order of 3.6 per 100 000 women per year at age 20, rising to 36 per 100 000 women per year at age 40 [4].

In most cases, stroke occurs as a separate event from an attack of migraine. Rarely, stroke has occurred during the course of a migraine aura, known as migrainous infarction. To confirm a diagnosis of migrainous infarction, the neurological deficit of the stroke must occur in the course of a typical migraine attack, and other causes of stroke must be excluded.

The cause remains uncertain. Regional cerebral blood flow studies have shown reduced cerebral blood flow during migraine aura. This has been considered to be sufficient to cause ischaemic focal neurological deficits. This view is supported by the results of magnetic resonance imaging studies which demonstrate white-matter lesions, thought to be ischaemic, in up to 40% of migraineurs.

Distinguishing between the focal symptoms of a migraine aura and the focal symptoms of a transient ischaemic attack is a matter of confusion for many doctors. This is discussed in details in Chapter 13.

Implications for treatment

Reducing risks is an important aspect of stroke prevention (Table 12.1). In young women, smoking is probably the greatest contributing factor. Primary care teams have a role in health education and should encourage all patients to stop smoking. Despite health risks, smoking is on the increase in young women. Other factors such as hypertension or diabetes mellitus should be identified and managed appropriately. If there is a strong family history of early stroke, familial disease should be sought. Combined oral contraceptives should be avoided by women with attacks of migraine with aura, who are at increased risk (see Chapter 10).

There is some clinical evidence that aspirin is effective in the prophylaxis of migraine with aura, although trial data are lacking. Certainly, patients at high risk of stroke could consider prophylactic aspirin to

Table 12.1 Risk factors for stroke.

Age ≥ 35
Diabetes mellitus
Family history of arterial disease ≤ 45 years
Hyperlipidaemia
Hypertension
Migraine
Obesity (body mass index > 30)
Smoking

decrease platelet aggregability. Vasoconstrictor drugs, particularly ergotamine, should be avoided.

Careful assessment is the key to successful management. Identification of the minority at particular increased risk of stroke and treatment of factors such as hypertension ot hypercholesterolaemia can reduce the likelihood of stroke occurring. Discriminatory questions can sometimes identify symptoms of an impending stroke but can also reassure those who are uncertain whether their symptoms are benign. Secondary prevention after a stroke is also important, again with assessment of risk factors which can be managed, and consideration of prophylactic aspirin.

References

1 Couch JR, Hassanein RS. Amitriptyline in migraine prophylaxis. *Arch Neurol* 1979; 36: 695–9.
2 Mathew NT, Saper JR, Silberstein SD *et al.* Migraine prophylaxis with divalproex. *Arch Neurol* 1995; 52: 281–6.
3 Medina JL, Diamond S. Migraine and atopy. *Headache* 1976; 15: 271–4.
4 Lidegaard O. Oral contraceptives, pregnancy and the risk of cerebral thromboembolism: the influence of diabetes, hypertension, migraine and previous thrombotic disease. *Br J Obstet Gynaecol* 1995; 102: 153–9.

12

CHAPTER 13

When it's not Migraine: Danger Signals, Tumours and Strokes

Although most headaches are benign, some headaches give rise to concern, often of a brain tumour or stroke. When patients consult with headache, correct diagnosis and reassurance, when appropriate, are essential to effective management.

Headache danger signals

When evaluating a patient with headache, the primary task is to exclude urgent, life-threatening causes of headache. Fortunately, the majority of headaches raise no cause for concern but the following symptoms and signs raise suspicion for urgent referral

On history

- Sudden onset of new severe headache, particularly if over age 50.
- Progressively worsening headache or associated symptoms over several days/weeks.
- Atypical neurological symptoms.
- New or persistent neurological deficit.
- Alteration in consciousness.
- Headache associated with nausea, vomiting and fever which cannot be attributed to causes such as colds or flu.
- Headaches triggered by exertion, coughing, bending or sexual activity.

These changes can occur in a patient with a long-standing history of primary headache who should be alerted to the development of new, or unusual, symptoms.

On examination

- Signs of toxic events, for example infection, haemorrhage.
- Severe hypertension.
- Neurological signs including papilloedema or haemorrhages on fundoscopy, neck stiffness, altered consciousness, or weakness.

Headache associated with intracranial pathology

Patients presenting with recent headaches should always prompt a high index of suspicion. Although the vast majority of patients have a benign form of headache, symptoms and signs should be carefully elicited to avoid missing the rare diagnosis of intracranial pathology.

Space-occupying lesions (Table 13.1)

The most common cerebral tumours in adults are metastatic and are associated with multiple lesions and widespread disseminated disease. Primary brain tumours are rare, with an annual incidence of 6 per 100 000 people. This amounts to an average of one patient every 10 years in a list of 2000 patients.

Headache is the sole presenting symptom in fewer than 10% of tumours. This is more likely to occur with fast-growing, more malignant tumours, especially posterior fossa tumours, in which headache is a symptom in up to 50% of cases. However, associated neurological symptoms soon follow as pressure affects brain structures. Slower growing, low-grade neoplasms only cause headache in about 5% of cases and are more likely to present with seizures. Frontal lobe tumours may be associated only with subtle personality changes prompting treatment for depression.

If the tumour is associated with raised intracranial pressure, the headache is typically subacute, non-pulsatile and worse on waking.

13

Table 13.1 Space-occupying lesions vs migraine.

	Brain tumour	Migraine
History	Months	Years
Attack frequency	Usually progressive	Intermittent
Pain	Deep steady dull ache	Throbbing
Site of pain	Unilateral and usually in the same place	Variable
Vomiting	Spontaneous and does not relieve headache	Associated with nausea and often relieves headache
Effect of movement/coughing/straining	Aggravates headache	Aggravates headache
Onset of symptoms	Wakes patient from sleep	Present on waking or develops during the day

Associated vomiting is spontaneous, without a build-up of nausea, and does not relieve the headache. It is exacerbated by any activity that can increase pressure, such as coughing, sneezing and bending. Symptoms are progressive, increasing in frequency and severity.

Mental state examination reveals personality changes, depression, memory loss, confusion and poor concentration. Bilateral papilloedema may be evident on fundoscopy.

Other focal neurological signs depend on the site of the lesion: lesions of the cerebral cortex produce seizures; lesions of the optic tract result in an homonymous hemianopia; lesions on cranial nerves produce cranial nerve palsies.

Stroke

Headache is a common premonitory symptom of both haemorrhagic and thrombotic stroke and can precede these events by days or weeks. Suspicion of stroke requires immediate investigation.

Haemorrhagic stroke, particularly subarachnoid haemorrhage, is less common than thrombotic stroke but is more often accompanied by localized headache. Headache is severe and instantaneous 'like being hit with a sledgehammer', associated with neck stiffness, photophobia and neurologic deficit. Fifty per cent of patients have a premonitory headache, with mild, intermittent symptoms. Rupture of an aneurysm is the most common cause or an underlying arteriovenous malformation may be found. Since aneurysms are more likely to leak when intracranial pressure is raised, onset during exertion is likely. Occasionally, examination reveals subhyaloid haemorrhages on fundoscopy. Computed tomography (CT) or lumbar puncture are diagnostic and are warranted in any patient who complains of the most severe headache ever, particularly if associated with exertion, straining or coitus.

Premonitory headaches associated with thrombotic strokes are often unilateral and throbbing, lasting for several hours. Age is the obvious factor to raise suspicion, particularly in the presence of symptoms and signs of cardiovascular disease. Early prophylaxis with low-dose aspirin can prevent further ischaemia developing.

Investigation: computed tomography or magnetic resonance imaging?

An increasing number of primary care physicians have direct access to imaging facilities. These investigations should be considered for patients with headache danger signals listed above. It is important to choose the correct initial investigation otherwise the diagnosis can be missed [1]. Magnetic resonance imaging (MRI) is expensive and patients find lying in such a confined space difficult to tolerate.

MRI is superior to CT in the detection of thrombotic but not haemorrhagic stroke. Cranial CT, without contrast and promptly performed, can distinguish cerebral haemorrhage from ischaemic stroke, as it will reveal fresh intracerebral blood, which appears white due to its iron content. A negative CT does not exclude intracerebral haemorrhage and, in these cases, lumbar puncture should be performed. MRI may miss fresh blood but an old bleed may be apparent after 1 or 2 weeks. Consequently, CT is recommended for stroke patients who need imaging in the first 48 h.

MRI is also best for imaging parenchymal brain infection and arteriovenous malformations.

MRI is often used to provide more detailed information following diagnosis of a suspected intracranial tumour by CT scan. MRI is superior to CT when imaging lesions in the region of the posterior fossa, axial tumours, the orbit and the paranasal sinuses, and demyelinating lesions.

Differences between migraine aura and thrombotic events (Table 13.2)

Doctors are often concerned about distinguishing between transient ischaemic attacks and migraine aura, particularly in older patients. Patients who have a long history of classical migraine are rarely a cause for concern. However, the natural history of migraine is such that attacks of migraine without aura can convert to attacks with aura with age, pregnancy or other hormonal triggers. In these circumstances, it is necessary to take a careful history to ensure symptoms are typical of migraine.

The diagnosis can be difficult since attacks of migraine aura can occur without an ensuing headache and headache is not uncommon in

13

Table 13.2 Focal symptoms not typical of migraine.

Rapid onset of symptoms
Longer duration of neurological symptoms
Visual symptoms
Monocular (amaurosis fugax)
Negative (black) scotoma
Sensory or motor disturbance affecting the whole of one side
of the body or lower limb only
Epilepsy
Loss of consciousness

cerebral ischaemia. Fortunately, certain features of the migraine aura can help distinguish between migraine and the focal neurological symptoms of cerebral ischaemia.

Progression of symptoms

The evolution of a migraine aura is slow, taking several minutes to spread to maximum distribution. In contrast, the motor/sensory spread of cerebral ischaemia is rapid, taking only seconds to move from the face to the hand, progressing rapidly down the trunk to affect the lower limb.

Symptoms

Visual symptoms

The visual symptoms of migraine are usually symmetrical, affecting one hemifield of both eyes, although subjectively they may appear to affect only one eye—if there is any doubt, patients should be asked to assess their next attack. A migrainous scotoma is typically positive (bright), starting as a small spot gradually increasing in size to assume the shape of a letter C, developing scintillating edges which appear as zigzags (fortifications—a term coined in the late 18th century because the visual disturbances resembled a fortified town surrounded by bastions). The aura usually starts at or near the centre of fixation, gradually spreading laterally, increasing in size over a period of 5–30 min. In contrast, thrombotic symptoms do not generally have the scintillating and spreading features of the visual aura of migraine and the visual loss is usually a monocular negative scotoma (black). Transient monocular blindness is *not* typical of migraine and prompts urgent investigation.

Sensory symptoms

Sensory symptoms are commonly positive, i.e. a sensation of pins and needles rather than numbness. In an ischaemic episode, a sense of numbness or 'deadness' is described. Migraine symptoms have a characteristic unilateral distribution affecting one arm, often spreading over several minutes proximally from the hand to affect the mouth and tongue—'cheiro-oral distribution'. This spread of paraesthesia to involve the tongue is typical of migraine aura and rarely seen in cerebrovascular attacks.

13

Past history of symptoms

Migraine auras usually follow a similar pattern with each attack, although the duration of aura may alter. Therefore, a long history of similar attacks, particularly if attack onset is in youth or early adult life, is typical of migraine. If aura symptoms suddenly change, further investigation may be warranted.

Reference

1   Armstrong P, Keevil SF. Magnetic resonance imaging—2: clinical uses. *BMJ* 1991; 303: 105–9.

13

CHAPTER 14

When it's not Migraine: Other Headaches

Having excluded sinister causes with a brief, but thorough, history and neurological examination, time taken to elicit a more careful history can reap benefits in short- and long-term management. When distinguishing migraine from other headaches, the simple rule of 'daily headaches are not migraine' applies (Table 14.1). The difficulty arises when several headaches coexist. This is often overcome by asking the patients 'How many different headaches do you have?' taking a separate headache history for each. Diary cards are also an invaluable aid to diagnosis (Fig. 14.1). Each type of headache follows a separate pattern, for example episodic attacks of migraine with increased headache severity and associated nausea will be superimposed on a background of less severe daily headache.

The International Headache Society (IHS) has developed a classification for headache disorders. These can be separated into primary headaches, such as migraine, tension-type headache and cluster headache, and headaches that are secondary to other conditions such as hangover or head injury (Table 14.2). The most common cause of non-migraine headache seen in general practice is tension-type headache. Medication-misuse headache is an increasingly common cause of secondary headache which can easily be prevented. Other headaches are identi-

Table 14.1 Daily headaches.

Common	Rare
Primary headaches	*Primary headaches*
Muscle contraction headache	Cluster headache
Tension headaches associated with stress/anxiety	Chronic paroxysmal hemicrania
Secondary headaches	*Secondary headaches*
Sinus infection	Headache associated with vascular
Medication-misuse headache	disorders, e.g. arteritis (< 55 years), dissection, arteriovenous malformation
	Headache associated with intracranial infection

15	Thu								
16	Fri	Mild	7 am	All day	No	No	Paracetamol	7 am	
17	Sat	Mild	7 am	All day	No	No	Paracetamol	7 am	
18	Sun	Mild	8 am	All day	No	No	Paracetamol	8 am	
19	Mon	Mild	7 am	All day	No	No	Paracetamol	7 am	
20	Tue	Moderate	7 am	All day	Yes	No	Paracetamol	7 am 1 pm	Late night
21	Wed	Mild	7 am	'til 6 pm	No	No	Paracetamol	7 am	
22	Thu	Mild	7 am	All day	No	No			
23	Fri	Mild	7 am	All day	No	No			
24	Sat	Severe	10 am		Yes	Yes	Paracetamol	10 am 1 pm	v. tired slept in
25	Sun	Severe			Yes	Yes			
26	Mon	Severe	↓	↓	Yes	No			
27	Tue	Mild	7 am	All day	Yes	No	Paracetamol	10 am	
28	Wed	Mild	7 am	'til 10 am	No	No	Paracetamol	7 am	
29	Thu	None			No	No			GOOD DAY
30	Fri	None			No	No			"
31	Sat	Mild	7 am	All day	No	No	Paracetamol	7 am	Hangover

Fig. 14.1 A diary card can aid diagnosis.

fied by their association with infections, metabolic disorders or structural disease.

Tension-type headache (Figs 14.2 & 14.3)

In clinical practice, two varieties of tension-type headache are seen: headaches related to local muscle pains, and headaches associated with depression and/or anxiety. The two can be distinguished by differences in the history and by response to medication (Table 14.3).

14

Table 14.2 Secondary headaches. Reproduced with permission from Rasmussen B. Epidemiology of headache. *Cephalalgia* 1995; 15: 45–68.

IHS code		%
5	Head trauma	4
6	Vascular disorders	1
7	Non-vascular cranial disorders	0.5
8	Substances or their withdrawal	3
8.1.4	Hangover	72
9	Non-cephalic infection	63
10	Metabolic disorder	22
11	Disorders of the cranium, neck, eyes	0.5–3
11.5	Sinuses	15
12	Cranial neuralgias	0.5

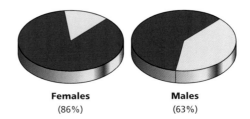

Females
(86%)

Males
(63%)

Fig. 14.2 Tension-type headache: 1-year prevalence. Based on data from Rasmussen BK. Epidemiology of headache. *Cephalalgia* 1995; 15: 45–68.

Local muscle pains (Fig. 14.4)

Most people have experienced the pain of aching muscles after unaccustomed exercise. The muscles feel sore and tender to touch. Lying in a hot bath or gentle massage often helps. The muscles of the head are

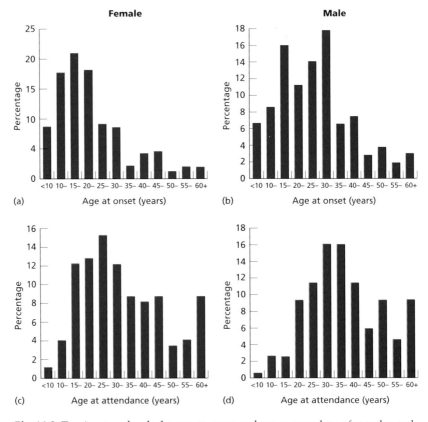

Fig. 14.3 Tension-type headache: age at onset and age at attendance for males and females. From MacGregor (unpublished data).

Table 14.3 Tension-type headache.

	Muscle contraction	Tension/depression
Age at onset	Any age, usually older	Any age
Frequency	Episodic or daily	Usually daily
Duration	Days to weeks	Continuous
Between attacks	Tender neck/shoulders muscles	Depressed
Headache	Localized Tender to touch	All-over pressure Band around the head Weight on the head
Associated symptoms	None	Mild if present
Affect	Normal	Depressed
General health	Well	Complains of being unwell but no specific symptoms
Use of acute medication	Episodic	Frequent, often daily
Effect of medication	Pharmacological response in 20–30 min with pain often returning after 3–4 h	Ineffective but many continue to take it daily. Differential diagnosis of medication-misuse headache

no different. Often the pain is localized, and patients can point to the site of pain, in contrast to the generalized pain of 'tension' headache.

Pain can be referred: pain in the temples may originate from the temporomandibular joints. Neck and shoulder muscle pains also give

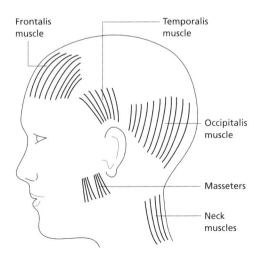

Frontalis muscle

Temporalis muscle

Occipitalis muscle

Masseters

Neck muscles

Fig. 14.4 Some muscles can give rise to headache.

rise to headaches especially in long-distance drivers or people sitting at a computer all day. Although analgesics may provide temporary relief within 30–45 min, they are only treating the symptoms and not the cause. Examination will reveal tense and tender neck, shoulder and/or jaw muscles but is otherwise normal. Effective management should be directed to treatment and prevention of the underlying physical basis using physical treatments such as exercise, physiotherapy, osteopathy and chiropractic, and paying attention to causative factors in the environment.

Tension headaches associated with depression/anxiety

Patients often describe this type of headache as a 'band around my head' or 'a weight pressing down on top of my head'. The history is typically vague. The pain is often generalized and present most of the time, typically worsening through the day. It may interfere with sleep particularly if the sufferer is depressed or anxious. Time is rarely lost from work but concentration may be poor. Pain killers have little effect although they may dull the pain for a couple of hours or so. Some patients continue frequent use of pain killers which can result in a secondary medication-misuse headache. Examination is essentially normal. Effective management is directed to treatment of the underlying cause, for example treatment of depression, stress management, etc. A course of antidepressants such as amitriptyline can be useful, particularly if sleep is affected. The initial dose should be low, for example 10 mg taken 2 h before bedtime, and gradually increased, if necessary. It is important to warn patients against overuse of analgesics as this can compound the problem.

14

Case study

Diana is 52 and works in a factory. She has had migraine without aura since her early twenties. She first consulted her doctor when she was 45 as the migraines had become more frequent, occurring monthly with her period, and lasting 3 days. These attacks were controlled with analgesics plus an antiemetic and a triptan. She still has occasional attacks of migraine, which respond to treatment. She now presents with a continuous headache, which she has had for several weeks. It is quite different from her previous attacks, as the pain is not so severe. She describes it as a tight feeling in her head, sometimes like a heavy weight on her head. There are no associated symptoms but she is having problems sleeping. She does not take any medication, as painkillers have not been effective. She admits to being worried about her husband as she thinks he may be having an affair. She starts to cry but quickly tries to regains composure. She is taking hormone replacement therapy to control menopausal symptoms. Physical examination is normal. The doctor asks Diana if she thinks she could be depressed. Diana admits that she does not feel on top of things and often bursts into tears. She discusses her fears about her husband, stating that she does not feel he could love her in her present state. The doctor prescribes a course of antidepressants, pointing out the expected early side-effects. She asks Diana to make a follow-up appointment.

Comment

Depression is a condition that frightens many patients, who think it is a sign of weakness. It can be helpful to point out the depression can be a chemical disorder, in which case antidepressants may help. Many patients stop treatment early because of side-effects, particularly sedation. This can be avoided by highlighting the need to continue treatment for several weeks before assessing negative and beneficial effects.

Medication-misuse headache (Fig. 14.5)

For most people, analgesics and other acute headache treatments are safe and effective. However, for a small percentage of patients the frequent use of acute treatments has a paradoxical effect on headache, perpetuating the cycle of pain rather than relieving it and contributing to a transformation from episodic to daily headaches [1]. This is thought to account for about 1% of the overall population, but up to 10% of patients attending specialist headache clinics.

This is not a new phenomenon; in 1957 a Swiss medical journal included a report on over-the-counter compounds containing phenace-

14

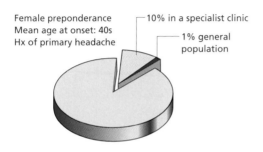

Fig. 14.5 Medication misuse headache.

tin as a cause of chronic headache. In the early 1980s, other researchers showed that other non-narcotic analgesics taken for 'instant relief' had a similar effect, even simple analgesics such as aspirin or paracetamol. The problem can be compounded by patients seeking relief by using stronger painkillers, often containing caffeine and codeine, which have addictive potential in their own right. Misuse of ergotamine and the triptans can also be associated with frequent headache [2,3].

The exact mechanism underlying medication-misuse headache is unknown but it is generally believed that a disturbance of central pain systems is involved. It is possible that the overuse of acute treatments could result in up- or down-regulation of specific pain receptors. It has been shown that 77% of patients with chronic daily headache overuse symptomatic drugs. Only patients who are prone to headaches develop this syndrome which is not seen in patients taking daily analgesics for reasons other than headache such as arthritis or back pain.

Identifying cases

Doctors can be alerted to patients who may be misusing acute treatments, before the patient seeks advice, by checking the repeat prescription system. If patients are repeatedly requesting the maximum allowance of analgesics or other acute migraine treatments, consider calling the patient in for an appointment.

History and examination (Table 14.4)

Typically the patient has a history of infrequent attacks of primary headaches. In the case of migraine, attacks rarely occur more than once or twice a month and are usually controlled adequately with simple analgesics or specific migraine treatments. Attacks may become more frequent, or the patient fears an impending attack and uses pre-emptive treatment with increasing frequency. Sometimes the process starts with the development of an additional non-migraine headache that is mistreated as migraine. Eventually, acute treatments may be taken most days, sometimes several times a day. Gradually, the headaches increase in frequency until they occur most days. Daily headache does not replace the episodic attacks and migraine can be superimposed. If the patient cannot differentiate the different headaches easily, use of a daily symptom diary card is invaluable.

On taking the history, the medication-misuse headache is worse when plasma levels of the drug are lowest, typically on waking. This pattern often raises the concern of a tumour headache but the symp-

Table 14.4 Differences between migraine and medication-misuse headache.

	Migraine	Medication misuse
Age at onset	Teens/twenties	Thirties/forties
Frequency	Episodic	Daily
Duration	2–72 h	All day unless Rx
Between attacks	'Fine'	Rarely free from symptoms
Headache	Often unilateral Severe Throbbing	All-over/diffuse Variable severity Dull
Associated symptoms	Nausea Vomiting Photo/phonophobia	Rarely present unless superimposed migraine
Affect	Normal between attacks	Flat 'Suppressed'
General health	Well	Tired Not coping
Use of acute medication	Episodic	Most days Often several different drugs Often on waking May be repeated during day
Effect of medication	Right medication effective	'Dulls' the pain

toms are not progressive. The pain is dull and constant but may wax and wane throughout the day. It is temporarily relieved (in many cases only partially) with acute headache treatments. Despite this lack of effect, patients often state that a migraine may develop unless they take treatment, perpetuating the cycle of medication misuse. Associated symptoms are few and mild, rarely affecting daily activities, although the patient may be depressed. Constipation and lethargy are common problems with frequent use of analgesics. Nausea, irritability, memory deficit and insomnia may also occur.

The examination is essentially normal in patients misusing analgesics or triptans. Patients misusing ergotamine may have symptoms of ergotamine toxicity, with reduced peripheral circulation, hypertension and cardiovascular disease, or even overt ergotism.

Treatment

The headache is resistant to alternative treatments, both drug prophy-

14

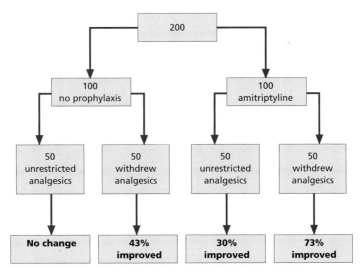

Fig. 14.6 Prophylaxis over 4/12. Based on data from Kudrow L. Paradoxical effects of frequent analgesic use. *Adv Neurol* 1982; 33: 335–41.

laxis and non-drug regimens, and the only effective management is to stop the patient from taking the drugs for at least 6–12 weeks. It is not possible to substitute alternative analgesics since these will have the same effect. Stopping acute treatments can either be with immediate withdrawal [4] or by gradual reduction of the amount of drug taken each day over several weeks. Withdrawal symptoms, consisting of excruciating headaches, nausea, vomiting, anxiety and insomnia, appear within 48 h and may last for up to 2 weeks. This is the time when most support is needed. Clinical studies show that up to 60% of patients who are withdrawn from acute treatments improve [5]. The addition of amitriptyline as a single night-time dose can aid recovery but only in combination with drug withdrawal (Fig. 14.6) [1]. Withdrawal should be done under doctor's supervision, as any other underlying causes of headache should be excluded.

Management of superimposed migraine can be a problem as effective treatment for these attacks is still necessary during drug withdrawal. Using a different route, or prescribing a drug with a different mechanism of action, can be an effective temporary measure. For example, if oral analgesics were being misused, acute migraine attacks could still be treated with analgesic and antiemetic suppositories or with triptans; if ergotamine or triptans were misused, suppositories are recommended. Obviously, caution is necessary to avoid misuse of these treatments.

If headaches persist several weeks after drug withdrawal, the diagnosis should be reassessed with history and examination. Further investigation may be indicated, and certainly if symptoms are progressive or if new symptoms develop.

Prevention

In clinical practice, medication-misuse headache may occur in any patient who has taken acute headache treatments regularly on more than 2 or 3 days a week for 3 months or more. Therefore, all patients should be counselled about appropriate use of medication, warning against the frequent use of analgesics. Non-migraine headaches should be diagnosed and managed appropriately. Prophylactic therapy should be considered if migraine attacks become frequent.

Case study

Denise is 46 and has had migraine without aura since childhood. She did not see a doctor about headaches until she was 42. At that time, she had had a continuous headache for 3 months. She had a stressful job as a teacher and was finding it difficult to cope with an increasing workload. The doctor she saw recommend simple analgesics which she started to take most days. The headaches became more of a problem and eventually she was forced to take early retirement. She was prescribed stronger painkillers, which she has continued to take. She makes an appointment with the new doctor, to get a repeat prescription. The doctor asks questions about the headaches, noting that Denise has attacks of migraine without aura about once a week which last for 1–2 days. In addition, she has daily headaches, worse on waking, with no associated symptoms. She is taking eight to 10 tablets of paracetamol and codeine most days, with a triptan for migraine. The pattern of symptoms and drug use have remained unchanged for the past couple of years. Examination is normal. The doctor expresses concern about the amount of medication that Denise is taking. Denise agrees, stating that she has tried to reduce the drugs but if she tries to stop taking them, she will get a migraine. The doctor discusses the problem that frequent use of acute drugs can aggravate headache. Denise says she is keen to stop taking so many drugs but does not know how to stop. The doctor helps her to draw up a gradual reducing programme and prescribes amitriptyline, to be taken at night. She sees Denise every week to assess her progress. After a couple of months, Denise is down to one painkiller a day. She has continued to use a triptan to treat migraine. She continues to progress over the next few months and stops the am-

14

itriptyline. Eventually she is only having migraine infrequently and the symptoms respond rapidly to simple analgesics.

Comment

Medication misuse headache often develops over several years, with the patient gradually increasing the dose and strength of medication taken. Many patients present with a picture of frequent migraine, failing to inform the doctor about daily headache. Although diary cards can be helpful, some patients will fail to record daily headaches unless specifically asked to record all symptoms. Often, it is not until several management strategies have been tried, all of which fail, that medication misuse is considered. A careful drug history, which may need to be requested on several occasions, will highlight the problem. Abrupt withdrawal of analgesics is the favoured technique but is not suitable for all. A gradual structured reduction in drug use over several weeks, regularly reviewed, is usually effective provided that the patient is motivated.

Other headaches

Most other headaches are associated with obvious disease and are rarely a cause of diagnostic difficulty. However, two specific headaches warrant a more detailed mention. Cluster headaches, although as rare as brain tumours, are often confused with migraine but require specific management. Headache associated with intracranial pathology, such as strokes or tumours, also merits inclusion as this type of headache is the one that most patients—and their doctors—fear.

14

Cluster headache (migrainous neuralgia) (Fig. 14.7)

Cluster headaches have an estimated prevalence rate of less than 1% (Fig. 14.8). The condition is a predominantly male disorder with a male/female ratio of 6:1. The age at onset is during the early 30s and the patient often smokes or has a history of smoking. A family history of cluster headache is rare. As the name suggests, attacks come in clusters once or twice a year lasting an average of 6–8 weeks. A few patients have chronic cluster headache with no periods of remission from attacks (Fig. 14.9). The underlying pathophysiology remains elusive.

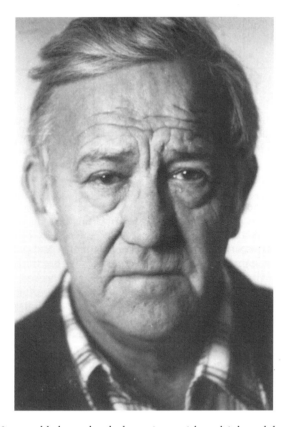

Fig. 14.7 A 62-year-old cluster headache patient, with multiple and deep furrows in forehead and face ('leonine' appearance). From Sjaastad O. *Cluster Headache Syndrome.* Philadelphia, WB Saunders, 1991, by permission of WB Saunders Company Limited, London.

14

History and examination

Although a 'leonine' appearance has been described, it is not often seen. The clinical history is characteristic and quite different from migraine. During a cluster period, patients experience an average of one to three attacks each day of very severe unilateral pain lasting between 20 and

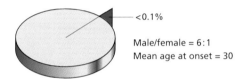

< 0.1%

Male/female = 6:1
Mean age at onset = 30

Fig. 14.8 Cluster headache: 1-year prevalence. Based on data from Rasmussen BK. Epidemiology of headache. *Cephalalgia* 1995; 15: 45–68.

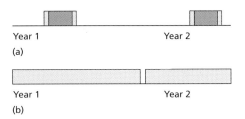

Fig. 14.9 Periodicity of cluster headache. (a) Episodic cluster headache. (b) Chronic cluster headache.

120 min. Attacks often wake the patient from sleep at the same time every night. The pain builds up rapidly to peak within a few minutes of onset. The headache always occurs on the same side during each cluster and is usually centred over one eye, which waters and appears bloodshot. The nostril on the affected side is blocked and there may be a discharge. The contralateral side is completely unaffected. The patient prefers to be left alone and paces up and down, often holding his head, rocking it back and forth. He may put pressure on the painful area or rub sufficiently hard to cause bleeding. The pain is so severe and intense that some patients become violent during an attack or repeatedly hit their heads. Symptoms subside rapidly but the area around the affected eye may feel 'bruised' between attacks.

Alcohol may trigger attacks but only during the cluster. Sublingual nitro-glycerine and histamine can also provoke attacks. No other triggers have been identified and avoidance of migraine triggers is irrelevant to management despite common practice. Apart from migraine, the differential diagnoses include trigeminal neuralgia, temporal arteritis or more rarely, phaeochromocytoma or chronic paroxysmal hemicrania.

Treatment

Treatment is aimed at reducing the frequency and severity of attacks during the cluster. It has no effect on the natural history of the condition. Side-effects and contraindications for the drugs recommended is discussed in the chapter on migraine management strategies.

Acute

Oral medication, unless the drug is rapidly absorbed, is rarely effective in the acute treatment of cluster headache, due to rapid onset and short duration of attacks.

Oxygen, provided the delivery rate is adequate, is safe and highly effective—provided patients are warned to keep well away from the cylinder when smoking! However, portable oxygen is an expensive option and most patients require additional ergotamine or a triptan to treat attacks away from home.

Oxygen. Ideally, 100% oxygen at 7 l/min, via facial mask for 10–20 min. The oxygen is available on prescription but a special regulator is necessary to achieve the high flow. The standard NHS regulators, usually supplied with a soft face mask, only deliver 28% oxygen at 2–4 l/min— an inadequate amount for treatment of cluster headache. A regulator and face mask, which allows delivery of up to 15 litres of oxygen per minute and up to 60% concentration, can be purchased from BOC Medical Gases. The mask should be firm and the holes taped over. Patients should be instructed to use the oxygen while sitting, leaning forward with the mask firmly over the face.

Ergotamine. One to three puffs from an ergotamine inhaler at onset of the attack. Maximum six puffs per 24 h, 15 per week.

Sumatriptan. One 6-mg subcutaneous injection at onset of the attack. Maximum two injections per 24 h. No weekly limit.

Prophylaxis

Prophylactic drugs are most effective when started early in the cluster. This is particularly the case for steroids. Verapamil is an effective first-line agent, but if there is no response to the maximum dose, it should be gradually withdrawn and an alternative prescribed. Prophylactic ergotamine can prevent attacks and, although recommended maximum weekly doses may be exceeded, this is rarely associated with problems provided its use is restricted to several weeks only. Lithium and methysergide should only be given with regular supervision by the doctor. Failure to respond to treatment warrants specialist referral. In extreme cases, surgical treatment may be considered.

14

Verapamil. Initially 40 mg twice daily increasing over 7–10 days to maximum 120 mg four times daily, stopping at an effective prophylactic dose. This should be continued for the usual duration of cluster, then gradually reduced over 1–2 weeks. If attacks break through, the dose should be increased until control is maintained and then reduced again at 2-weekly intervals.

Ergotamine (not for chronic use). One-half to one Cafergot suppository (1–2 mg) 1–4 h before expected attacks, for example use at bedtime for night-time attacks. This should be continued only for the expected duration of cluster and no longer than 6–8 weeks if tolerated. It should be stopped if vascular insufficiency or other signs of ergotism develop.

Steroids. Prednisolone 20 mg three times daily reducing over 10–14 days.

Methysergide. One to four milligrams daily in divided doses—maximum 6 mg daily. If used for chronic cluster headache, a 1-month break is necessary for every 6 months of use to prevent the rare possibility of retroperitoneal fibrosis.

Lithium. Occasionally used but regular blood levels are required. The usual dose is 800–1200 mg to give plasma levels of ≈ 1 mmol/l.

Case study

Tom is a 32-year-old mechanic. Over the last 2 years he has had bouts of daily headaches with each bout lasting a couple of weeks. His doctor thought they were sinus problems and prescribed antibiotics. He is back in the surgery and has an appointment with the trainee. He tells the doctor that he was free from symptoms for over 1 year but for the last week he has been woken up by the headaches at about 1 AM every morning. He says that the pain is so intense that he has to get up. He paces about the room, or rocks back and forth in a chair. The pain only affects the left side, never the right. His left eye waters and his nose runs from the left side. He describes his head as being cut in two with one side affected and the other side normal. The pain lasts about an hour and a half and then quickly subsides. His left temple feels 'bruised' between attacks. There are no other associated symptoms. He says that he avoids alcohol when he has these attacks as a drink can trigger a headache during the day. He admits to smoking 30 cigarettes a day. Painkillers have no effect. The doctor recognizes cluster headache and prescribes verapamil for prophylaxis and oxygen for acute treatment. Tom is given instructions how to use the oxygen mask and is advised not to smoke anywhere near the oxygen cylinder. Subcutaneous sumatriptan is prescribed for Tom to use to treat attacks at work.

Comment

Cluster headache can go unrecognized for many years, often mis-

14

diagnosed as sinusitis. The unilaterality and severity of symptoms, in addition to noting that the patient is woken from sleep by pain, confirms the diagnosis of cluster headache. Although little is known about the condition and there is no cure, effective management can reduce morbidity.

References

1 Kudrow L. Paradoxical effects of frequent analgesic use. *Adv Neurol* 1982; 33: 335–41.
2 Wainscott G, Volans G, Wilkinson M. Ergotamine induced headaches. *BMJ* 1974; 2: 742.
3 Gaist D, Tsiropoulos I, Sindrup SH *et al.* Inappropriate use of sumatriptan: population based register and interview study. *BMJ* 1998; 316: 1352–3.
4 Hering R, Steiner TJ. Abrupt withdrawal of medication in analgesic-abusing migraineurs. *Lancet* 1991; 337: 1442–3.
5 Baumgartner C, Wesely P, Bigot C, Maly J, Holzner F. Long-term prognosis of analgesic withdrawal in patients with drug-induced headaches. *Headache* 1989; 29: 510–4.

14

CHAPTER 15

Migraine in the Workplace

Migraine is most prevalent between the ages of 25 and 55 with a signifi-cant, but poorly recognized, effect on employment. Direct costs of migraine, related to diagnosis and management, are low leading to the mistaken belief that migraine is not an important condition to recognize or treat. However, the indirect costs arising from lost productivity can be enormous. Indirect costs are met by the economy so what relevance are these figures to general practice? The point is that migraine is increasingly recognized as a public health issue with absence from work an important problem (Fig. 15.1). The consequence is that the burden of identification and management of migraine will be shared between occupational health and general practice.

Identifying migraine at work

Until recently, migraine was rarely considered to be a problem affecting employment. However, several studies have identified a high prevalence of migraine in working populations, often inadequately treated. Why has this problem not been recognized in the past? There are several possible reasons. First, the social stigma of migraine has meant that many people state other reasons for taking sick leave. Secondly, an increasing female workforce has brought more migraine into the workplace.

Several studies have been undertaken in the UK to assess migraine at work. Three of the more recent ones are discussed.

A study of employees in a chemical industry research and commercial centre revealed migraine prevalence of 23% in women and 12% in men [1]. Attacks typically lasted about 13 h with an average of eight

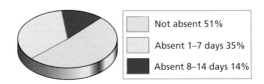

Not absent 51%

Absent 1–7 days 35%

Absent 8–14 days 14%

Fig. 15.1 Absence rates from work of migraineurs in the previous year. Based on data from Rasmussen BK. Epidemiology of headache. *Cephalalgia* 1995; 15: 45–68.

and a half attacks each year. Forty-two per cent had never sought medical advice regarding headaches and most used over-the-counter medication.

Similarly, a study of migraine in employees of an NHS Trust hospital in Hull undertaken in 1994 revealed that 158 of 1903 employees (8.3%) could be confirmed as having migraine [2]. A further 220 (11.6%) fulfilled three-quarters of the International Headache Society criteria, used to make the diagnosis. This means that nearly 20% of the respondents experienced disabling headaches. Prevalence was significantly greater in females. Compared with the earlier study, migraine was more frequent, averaging 16 attacks per year lasting 24 h. Migraine sufferers lost an average of 2 days from work each year due to their attacks. Reduced efficiency, estimated by number of equivalent days that would be lost if they were unable to work, increased this figure to 7.5 days. The estimated financial cost to the Trust, which employs a staff of 4200, through lost productivity was over £110 000 each year. Seventy-eight per cent were using only over-the-counter medication despite reporting significant impact of migraine on their lives. Only 40% of those identified with migraine had consulted a doctor in the previous 3 months, mostly contacting their GP, although a few used the occupational health service.

A more recent study in a Liverpool NHS Trust was undertaken in 1997 [3]. The results showed that 21% of respondents could be classified as having migraine, 60% of whom had not previously been diagnosed. The average frequency was 10 attacks per year, each lasting up to 17 h. Migraine sufferers lost about 3 days a year from work because of attacks. Although around half of respondents with regular headaches had consulted their GP, of concern is the finding that three-quarters of these had not continued to see their doctor and did not even collect repeat prescriptions.

The message from these three studies is clear. Despite a high prevalence of migraine in the workplace, particularly affecting women, medical advice is rarely sought and use of medication is suboptimal. The result is not only unnecessary individual disability, but also significant financial implications from lost productivity. Occupational health departments have an important role in identifying the problem as well as providing education and advice. Much of the information in this book can be put to use by occupational health staff. There is scope for educating both employees and their employers. Patients often comment that they are concerned that their job may be at stake if their employers find out that they have migraine. Better education of all parties involved could eliminate such fears. Raising the profile of migraine as a condi-

15

tion with an organic, rather than psychological, basis and for which there are effective treatments, has the potential markedly to destroy the numerous myths that surround the condition and improve working relationships. But to help employees with migraine, they have to be identified. Pre-employment and periodic medical assessments could be used to identify migraineurs. Once diagnosed, migraineurs experiencing attacks at work are more likely to seek treatment. If treated at work, they are more likely to return to work the same day rather than go home. Improvements in the working environment could be considered if relevant triggers such as noise or inadequate breaks from work are identified.

Case study

'I gave up work 2 years ago because, at that time, I was getting migraine every 8–10 days. There is no doubt that I was suffering from stress, not just because of the content of work, although it was a stressful job, but because of lack of understanding from colleagues and my employer. I had managed to cope in the past because I could predict my migraines to some extent. Then came a time when they became so frequent that I couldn't cope. People couldn't understand how I could just have a couple of days off work and then go back to work as if nothing had happened. Comments were made to me like 'Oh, have you had a nice day off?'. It hurt and I became very depressed. I could no longer function properly at work. Every time I had a day or 2 days off, the work would be building up. I was letting my colleagues down and I was letting my employer down. In the end it just became too much for me and, although I didn't want to, I had to resign.'

15

Comment

This patient lacked support from all parties concerned. She felt guilty about letting her colleagues and employer down, but the concern about missed work through migraine became an added trigger. An occupational health physician could have offered her support through the period of exacerbation of migraine, removing work pressures. Education of the employer and colleagues could have resulted in a more empathetic attitude and removed her sense of isolation. An interested and knowledgeable GP could provide her with a suitable management strategy. Effective acute treatment, and perhaps also prophylaxis, may enable her to continue work. It could also alleviate her fear of having an attack. Once through the crisis, triggers could be tackled and drug treatment adapted as indicated. She could have kept her job having created minimal burden to her employers.

Attacks at work

What about the employee who develops an attack while at work? Studies in specialist migraine clinics have shown the value of early medication and rest. This combination can often enable a rapid return to work within a few hours. Of 310 patients attending the City of London Migraine Clinic for acute treatment in 1976, 90% were either symptom-free or only had slight residual headache after 4 h [4]. All were given a combination of metoclopramide and an effervescent analgesic. In addition, 60% had taken a sedative and 10% took ergotamine. The study showed that those patients who slept recovered more quickly than those who did not. Obviously, acute treatment is not sufficient in itself. Providing a quiet, darkened area to rest can make a substantial difference.

Disability

Some patients seek advice about registering as disabled because of frequent migraine. To be classified under the Disability Discrimination Act (1995) a condition must be substantial and permanent. Since migraine is a condition which fluctuates, improves in later life, and usually shows some response to acute or prophylactic treatments, it is difficult to justify a claim of permanent disability. In such cases, there are usually other factors to consider, such as personal, work or social stresses, and even misdiagnosis. Workplace adjustment might be required in terms of changing lighting or temperature.

There are certain occupations which preclude migraineurs because of safety factors, such as commercial airline pilots and aerial climbers.

15

Occupational health meets general practice

Occupational health physicians cannot manage migraine alone. However, the above studies highlight the extent to which employees identified as having migraine lack contact with their GP. Although it may be necessary to administer acute treatments in the workplace, the responsibility for continuing migraine treatment usually falls to the GP. Migraine is no longer a condition that sufferers should expect to live with. Advances in our understanding of migraine and the development of specific drugs means that patients, friends, family, employers and even the government are putting increasing pressure on doctors to provide information and effective treatments. Managing migraine is a challenge that can, and should, be met in general practice.

References

1 Mountstephen AH, Harrison RKA. study of migraine and its effects in a working population. *Occup Med* 1995; 45: 311–7.
2 Clarke CE, MacMillan L, Sondhi S, Wells NEJ. Economic and social impact of migraine. *Q J Med* 1996; 89: 77–84.
3 Johnson G. The pain barrier. *Occup Health* 1997 (November): 16–20.
4 Wilkinson M, Williams K, Leyton M. Observations on the treatment of an acute attack of migraine. *Res Clin Stud Headache* 1978; 6: 141–6.

15

CHAPTER 16

Common Questions and Answers

Any person with an ailment has a thirst for knowledge about their condition. Information about migraine is increasingly available to the general public in magazines, health columns of newspapers, even the Internet. These are valuable sources of general information but do not replace advice from healthcare professionals. Primary care physicians have the advantage of being able to provide answers that are specific to each patient.

Many of the following questions have been provided by members of the Migraine Action Association and patients attending the City of London Migraine Clinic. Suggested replies follow each question.

About migraine

What is migraine? Migraine is more than just a headache. Changes in the chemistry of the brain cause subtle symptoms in mood or behaviour several hours before the headache even starts. About 30% of people also experience more specific neurological symptoms, typically affecting vision. Other symptoms, such as 'pins and needles' starting in the fingers of one hand, which gradually spread up the arm and into the face, may also occur. These events are known as an 'aura', which lasts about 10–30 min and is usually rapidly followed by headache. The headache of migraine is associated with nausea and/or vomiting, dislike of light and sound, sensitivity to smells and difficulty concentrating. These symptoms are often described as a 'power cut', making it difficult for the individual to continue with normal daily activities during an attack. However, they rarely last longer than 3 days after which normal function is restored. Research suggests that many of these symptoms are due to changes in brain levels of a chemical known as serotonin, or 5 hydroxytryptamine (5HT).

What happens in my brain during an attack? For centuries it was believed that the migraine aura was caused by constriction of blood vessels in the part of the brain responsible for processing vision. The headache was thought to be due to subsequent swelling of blood vessels in the brain. Certainly, the chemical known to be released during

16

migraine, serotonin, has powerful effects on the size of blood vessels. However, recent research suggests that the brain becomes more excitable during migraine, affecting the nerves involved in pain. It is thought that changes in the size of blood vessels are a response to these changes in the nervous system. Eventually the brain settles down and the attack subsides. The whole process usually takes 1–3 days.

Can frequent attacks cause any permanent damage? There is limited evidence to suggest that having frequent attacks of migraine causes any permanent damage to the brain. One of the features of migraine is that the symptoms are completely reversible. Migraineurs are usually fit and well between attacks, unless they have other specific medical or psychiatric problems. Some physicians even argue that migraine may be protective, by forcing the individual to withdraw from a build-up of stimuli, which could otherwise be potentially harmful to the body. However, serious conditions such as stroke can produce neurological symptoms which may, rarely, be mistaken for migraine, and vice versa. Fortunately stroke is very rare in the age group who most suffer from migraine but it is important that any change in migraine symptoms is checked out.

Why do I get migraine? It is probable that everyone can have migraine at some time. However, different people have different migraine 'thresholds'. This 'threshold' is probably inherited and represents the level at which migraine can be triggered. If a sufficient number of different internal and environmental triggers build up to reach this threshold, an attack is initiated. This explains why an individual does not always get an attack in similar situations—perhaps the threshold fluctuates, or the number or power of triggering factors is different.

What causes migraine? The triggers for migraine are many and varied. They differ between individuals and they differ between attacks. The commonest trigger factor, particularly in children, is hunger or insufficient food. Strenuous exercise can also trigger attacks, although regular exercise can help to prevent attacks. In women, hormonal fluctuations associated with the menstrual cycle can provoke migraine. It is unusual for a single factor to trigger attacks. More commonly, migraine results from a build-up of several trigger factors over a period of time. This means that the triggers are not always as obvious as they seem. For example, migraine occurring at the time of menstruation may result from a build-up of late nights and missed meals before the final trigger of menstruation crosses the migraine 'threshold' triggering

16

attacks. Although menstruation would seem to be the obvious trigger, regular meals and a better pattern of sleep could have prevented the build-up and thus the individual would remain below the attack threshold.

Can migraine be cured? There is no known cure for migraine. However, a great deal can be done to lessen the impact of migraine by providing effective acute treatments for migraine, identifying and avoiding triggering factors, and using preventative treatments when necessary. This can make the change from a condition that is out of control to one which is back in the patient's control.

Will I have migraine for the rest of my life? Migraine typically starts during the teens and twenties, although even young children can develop migraine. However, the majority of people cope with migraine in their youth. It is not until they reach their late thirties/early forties that migraine becomes a problem sufficient for them to seek medical advice. This is particularly the case for women who have the added trigger of hormonal problems at this time of life. In both sexes the frequency of migraine reduces in later life, usually after the age of 55. A few individuals continue to have frequent attacks although these are often complicated by the onset of other headaches or medical problems. Treating these conditions will usually help the migraine.

Will attacks always be this frequent? The frequency of attacks can vary considerably over time. Studies show that most people experience periods when they are free of migraine which can last between 2 and 10 years. Other times, attacks may occur frequently over several months.

Preventing migraine

Can migraine be prevented? Both non-drug treatments and drugs can be used to prevent migraine. In most cases, treatments reduce the frequency and severity of attacks rather than abolish them entirely. Drug treatments are usually considered when attacks are not adequately controlled with acute therapies alone and/or attacks prevent the individual from leading a normal life.

Is there anything I can do to prevent attacks without taking drugs? Yes. One method is to identify and avoid potential trigger factors. This can halve the frequency of migraine—as successful as many of the preventative drugs used in migraine. However, identifying relevant

16

triggers requires motivation and can be time consuming as triggers are not always obvious. Many patients favour alternative approaches such as relaxation techniques, physiotherapy, acupuncture, and osteopathy. These can be successful, particularly when muscle tension in the neck and shoulders is associated with migraine. Other treatments include herbal treatments and homeopathy. These are often confused with one another but are quite separate treatments. Herbal treatments such as feverfew are taken in doses that have similar effects to more orthodox drugs. In many cases, herbal treatments and orthodox medicines work in similar way. For example, feverfew has effects on the body that are very similar to aspirin. The practice of homeopathy is quite different, using specific remedies to treat all the different ailments of the individual. This means that two people with similar attacks but with other different problems will receive different treatments. For these reasons, it is important that patients consult qualified herbalists and homeopaths, rather than buying treatments from a health food shop. Since some herbs and remedies can interact with standard drugs, it is important that the GP knows about *all* treatments that are taken.

I have been told that there are many possible triggers for migraine attacks. How can I identify mine? Many people read about all the different migraine triggers and try to avoid them all, often without much success. The only way to identify relevant triggers is to keep an attack diary and a trigger diary over several months. On the attack diary, record all headaches and migraines when they occur, including the time of onset. To keep a trigger diary, buy a small notebook and make a record of a typical day's routine, including meal times, travel, work and leisure activities, etc. Every evening, record any differences to the usual routine. Also run through a list of typical migraine triggers and record any that happened that day. Note any unusual changes in mood or behaviour as these may be prodromal, or warning, symptoms. Some of these, particularly food and chocolate cravings, are often confused with triggers. After about 3 months, compare the attack and trigger diaries. It may be possible to identify a build-up of different triggers preceding attacks, for example frequent missed meals, disrupted sleep, work stresses, etc. By being aware of a potential build-up of triggers, it is often possible to compensate by taking extra care to minimize them in the future.

I have given up cheese, chocolate, citrus fruits, coffee and red wine but this has not made any difference to the frequency or severity of my migraine. Why? Although these are commonly cited as migraine triggers, in practice avoidance of these foods appears to make little difference

16

for the majority of patients. The minority who are sensitive to these foods will already be aware that ingestion is rapidly followed by migraine on every occasion and therefore already avoid them. For most migraineurs, the most important food trigger is lack of food. Provided regular meals are eaten, most foods can be eaten in moderation.

Can I stop my migraines by following an exclusion diet/cutting out certain foods from my diet? If a particular food is a suspect trigger, it can be eliminated from the diet for several weeks and then reintroduced. If multiple foods are suspected, it is best to seek medical advice before embarking on a strict diet as severe deficiencies can result.

I often think that my migraine might be caused by allergy. Is there somewhere I can go to find out? Allergy and migraine is a contentious issue. An allergic response can be assessed with simple tests. However, it is unlikely that migraine is caused by a true allergic response. Intolerance to certain foods has been implicated in migraine but this is much more difficult to test. Numerous techniques are available assessing hair and blood samples, although their reliability is questioned. Identification and management of food intolerance is based on restricting diet followed by gradual reintroduction of foods, as mentioned above.

I'd like to get fit but every time I start an exercise programme, I wake up next day with a migraine. What can I do? Studies show that fit people are less likely to have problems with migraine. Regular exercise has numerous benefits for body and mind. Unfortunately, getting fit can make things worse before they get better. Overenthusiastic erratic exercise causes stiff, aching muscles and may trigger attacks. This is no reason to avoid exercise. Unnecessary pain can be avoided if exercise is regular and graded to initial fitness. Stretching exercises and the beginning and end of a work-out can ease muscle tension, as can a hot bath or sauna. Deep heat creams or heat pads are also useful. An exercise programme is often initiated at the same time as a new diet. Inadequate nutrition can act as an additional trigger. It is important to eat sensibly and not to 'crash' diet.

16

I travel a lot for work but find that long plane trips inevitably trigger migraine. What can I do? Travelling is a common trigger for migraine for several reasons. First, there is the stress of preparing for a trip—clearing the desk, tidying the house, packing, etc. Then there is the stress of travelling—heaving suitcases, missing meals, coping with lack of sleep and jet-lag, climate changes, etc. Flying is associated with specific problems of reduced oxygen in the circulating air, dehydration, erratic mealtimes and sitting in a cramped seat for several hours. Advance planning can help. Take some snacks to eat, avoid alcohol, take bottled still water and drink plenty of fluids, and walk around the plane.

Diagnosing migraine

I get quite bad 'sick' headaches every month. Could it be migraine? Many people do not realize that their 'sick' headaches or 'bilious' attacks are migraine. Episodic headaches associated with nausea and sensitivity to light, which last between several hours and 3 days, are probably migraine.

My friend said that I can't have migraine because my vision isn't affected. Is this true? Even some doctors mistakenly believe that you have to have an 'aura' to diagnose migraine. Seventy per cent of migraine attacks are 'sick' headaches with no preceding aura.

I don't get many headaches but I get attacks of funny vision/numbness. Could this be migraine? In about 1% of attacks the aura of migraine occurs without an ensuing headache. This usually only happens in people who have had typical attacks of migraine aura with headache in the past. It is more common with advancing age. Provided the symptoms are typical of migraine aura, there is no need for any investigations. However, investigations may be necessary to rule out other causes if aura without headache develops for the first time in an older person, who has no history of migraine.

I get frequent attacks of migraine but why does no one find anything wrong with me when they examine me? One factor in diagnosing migraine is that a physical examination is normal. This is because the symptoms of migraine are due to changes in brain chemistry, which return to normal when the attack is over. There is no structural problem and hence, nothing to find on examination.

My friend saw a specialist about her headaches and had to have many tests, including a brain scan. But my GP just gave me a physical and told me I had migraine and didn't need a scan. Why not? Migraine is usually diagnosed from a description of typical attacks in the absence of physical signs. In most cases, no further investigations are necessary. But there are all sorts of reasons why tests and brain scans might be done. First, there may be doubt that the headaches are migraine, and

16

other causes need to be excluded. Secondly, many specialist centres are also research centres. Many tests and scans will be undertaken as part of specific research projects and not because of any medical need.

I suffer from two or three migraines every week. Could I have 'cluster migraine'? Although the term 'cluster migraine' is sometimes used, it is meaningless as it confuses two, quite separate, conditions: migraine and cluster headache. Migraine is an episodic headache with complete freedom from symptoms between attacks. Symptoms last for about 1–3 days. The frequency of attacks varies but may average one attack every 2–8 weeks. Cluster headache is rare, with several differences that distinguish it from migraine. Attacks may occur daily, often at night, for several weeks. The headaches last between 1 and 2 h, always affecting the same side of the head. The distinction is important as treatment for each condition is quite different. Patients reporting several 'migraines' each week need to be carefully assessed. Most commonly, the patient has migraine but has developed an additional headache. Sometimes they may be reporting recurrence of migraine related to triptan use. Alternative acute treatment may be indicated for future attacks. In other cases, frequent 'migraine' attacks are associated with misuse of acute medications, when analgesics, ergots or triptans are taken regularly on more than 2 days a week (see below).

Heredity

Will I pass migraine on to my children? The question of inheritance in migraine is complex. It appears that certain genes may be involved in migraine, and these may be associated with inheriting the migraine 'threshold'. This means that a person with the migraine genes is more susceptible to migraine triggers than a person without the genes. However, it is clear that genes are not the sole factor responsible for migraine. Environmental factors also play an important role.

16

Comorbidity

Whenever I get migraine, I always temporarily lose part of my sight. Could it become permanent? Permanent loss of vision is not an uncommon fear in people who have migraine aura, who often worry that they are having a stroke. However, the typical gradually developing visual symptoms of migraine are quite different to symptoms of stroke. It is extremely rare for visual loss to become permanent in migraine, especially in the absence of other risk factors for stroke.

Am I more likely to have a stroke? The majority of studies suggest that stroke is slightly more likely to occur in migraineurs although a few studies show a reduced risk of stroke. Certainly, migraine does appear to be an independent risk factor for ischaemic stroke in young women. However, the absolute risk is very small, with stroke affecting fewer than 6 out of a 100 000 women at the age of 20. The problem with studying a link between stroke and migraine is that stroke is very rare in the age group that suffer migraine. However, certain risk factors, such as smoking, particularly in women who also take the combined oral contraceptive pill, may slightly increase the risk of stroke. The risk of stroke due to smoking is much greater than the risk due to migraine so the obvious answer is to stop smoking.

Am I more likely to have a brain tumour? There is no evidence to suggest that people with migraine are at greater risk of developing a brain tumour than other healthy individuals. Brain tumours are rare— the average GP will see only one patient with a brain tumour every 10 years.

Am I more likely to have depression? There is some evidence that depression and migraine are linked. The chemical implicated in migraine, serotonin, is also involved in depression. Consequently, several treatments used in migraine and depression are the same.

Medication

The medication prescribed to relieve the pain of my migraine leaves my feeling nauseous and unwell. Is this normal? Are there other treatments I can try? Since nausea is a common symptoms of migraine, it is not always easy to distinguish between side-effects of drugs and symptoms of the attack. However, some drugs are known to aggravate nausea, particularly ergotamine and dihydroergotamine. Nausea can also occur after taking triptans but the effect is usually short-lived. If medication is the cause, symptoms will start when the drug is absorbed into the body. In the case of oral medication, this takes about 20–60 min. If nausea is a problem, antisickness drugs such as domperidone or metoclopramide can be prescribed. These drugs are compatible with most other migraine treatments.

My doctor gave me some antisickness tablets to take with painkillers for my migraine even though I don't get sick. Why? The stomach shuts down during a migraine attack, which means that oral medication may

16

not be absorbed into the body. Some antisickness drugs, such as domperidone and metoclopramide, help to reverse this shut-down. This can make medication more effective, avoiding the need for stronger drugs.

My doctor gave me some tablets to take when I have an attack but they don't seem to work, why not? The answer is essentially similar to the above. Taking an additional drug to aid absorption can solve the problem. However, it is important that tablets are taken as early as possible in a migraine attack. Many patients worry about taking migraine medication when they are not sure if they have a true attack. The answer is to try simple painkillers. These will work for a 'normal' headache. If they have not had any effect in 1 h then it is appropriate to take more specific migraine drugs. This advice should only be followed for infrequent headaches. Headaches occurring more often than once or twice a week require more specific management. For many, it is a matter of trial and error until the right treatment, or combination of treatments/ lifestyle changes, is found. Drugs prescribed for migraine in one individual may not work for a different person, even if the migraine appears the same. Some drugs may be dangerous if given to the wrong person. Go back to the doctor if the treatment is not effective and resist the temptation to try a friend's 'miracle' drug without medical advice.

I'm so sick with my migraines that I can't keep down any tablets. Is there anything else I can take? There are several alternatives to tablets. Analgesics and antisickness medications are available as suppositories. Ergotamine is available as a suppository and by inhalation. Dihydroergotamine is only given in the UK as a nasal spray. Sumatriptan can be prescribed a nasal spray or by self-injection. In some countries it is also available as a suppository. Nasal sprays of other triptans will be available in the near future. More novel methods of taking migraine drugs, such as a rapidly dissolving wafer, are being developed to improve absorption and efficacy.

16

I've been using a triptan for several years and it is very effective. The leaflet that comes with the tablets says I shouldn't take it if I'm over 65. Will I have to stop taking it? The triptans constrict the blood vessels in the head that are dilated in migraine, hence their effect. However, the concern is that blood vessels, such as those in the heart, are also affected. This is not a problem for young, fit, healthy individuals. The concern is that as we age, our blood vessels fur up, like a kettle. This is known as atherosclerosis and increases the risk of heart disease and stroke by narrowing the blood vessels. Drugs that further narrow blood vessels should be avoided. Obviously, some people are more at risk of atherosclerosis than others but it is not always easy to identify who is affected. Hence the recommendation that older people should avoid triptans.

My doctor gave me tablets to take every day to prevent attacks but it hasn't made any difference. Why not? There are several different reasons why preventative drugs taken each day are not effective. Some drugs take a few weeks before they start to take effect, so perhaps they have not been taken for long enough. The dose may need to be increased, as many doctors start with very low doses to reduce side-effects. Have several doses been missed? It can be difficult to remember to take medication several times a day. If the drug has been taken properly and in an adequate dose for several weeks but is still not working, it is worth trying a different drug. If no drug works, the diagnosis may be wrong. If no obvious cause is found, it is often the case that preventative drugs fail because the patient is misusing acute treatments and taking them too often. Reducing the amount of acute medication taken will usually reduce the frequency of migraine without the need for preventative drugs.

What side-effects can I expect from my medication? All effective drugs have side-effects. Not all are unpleasant and some can even be beneficial. For example, sedative side-effects can promote sleep when disrupted sleep is a migraine trigger. Your doctor or pharmacist can give you information about the expected side-effects of the drugs you are taking.

I'm not happy about taking drugs every day to prevent attacks. Are they addictive? None of the drugs commonly used for migraine prevention has addictive properties. However, when a person stops the medication, doctors usually recommend that the dose is gradually reduced. This is particularly helpful when the individual is concerned that the migraine will suddenly come back when the drug is stopped.

How long will I have to keep taking tablets every day to prevent migraine? Will I have to take them for the rest of my life? Most preventative drugs for migraine are taken only for a few months to break the cycle of frequent attacks. This is usually adequate, although if attacks return as the dose is reduced, it may be necessary to return to the original dose for a further few months. If drugs are taken for too long, side-effects can build up and create additional problems. This may be why

16

stopping preventative drugs is also associated with improvement! Courses of preventative drugs may need to be repeated if attacks become more frequent.

I'm not depressed but my doctor has prescribed antidepressants for my migraine. Why? Few drugs used in migraine are exclusive to migraine. Antidepressants, particularly amitriptyline, are commonly used to prevent migraine. They have an effect on serotonin, a chemical found in the brain that has been implicated in migraine.

My blood pressure is normal but my doctor has prescribed the same drug that my mother takes for her blood pressure. Why? Several research studies have shown that certain drugs used to treat blood pressure also effectively prevent migraine. The reason why these drugs are effective for migraine is not known. It is unlikely that it is anything to do with their effect on blood pressure as the low doses used in migraine are much lower than those needed to treat hypertension.

My doctor prescribed some tablets called Deseril (methysergide) which work really well. I've been taking them for 6 months and now I've been told I have to stop them for a month. Why? Methysergide is probably the most effective drug for preventing migraine. However, it is usually reserved for patients who have unsuccessfully tried other methods of preventing attacks and whose headaches are of such severity or frequency that their lives are severely disrupted. This is because long-term use of methysergide has been linked to a condition called fibrosis. This very rare condition can affect the kidneys, lungs and heart. This has only been reported in patients who have taken methysergide continuously and is not reported to occur if a regular break is taken from the drug. Therefore, it is recommended that methysergide is stopped for at least 1 month after every 6 months of treatment.

16

My doctor prescribed propranolol but the chemist gave me Inderal—is this OK? All drugs are known by several names. There is the chemical name, the generic name, and the brand name. For example, propranolol is the generic name and Inderal is a brand name of the same drug.

I'm taking tablets every day to prevent migraine but I don't always remember to take them. What should I do if I miss a dose? It depends how often you need to take the tablets. If you need to take them three times a day, and frequently miss doses, it may be more appropriate to ask about less frequent regimens; some drugs are available in long-acting, once-daily doses. If you forget to take a tablet that you are meant to take once or twice a day and are only a few hours late, take it immediately. If the next dose is due soon, skip the missed dose completely, but try to be more careful about taking future doses on time. Drugs cannot be effective when they are left in the bottle.

I can guarantee that I'm going to get a migraine when I have a long car journey or a special occasion that I've been looking forward to. Is there anything I can take to stop the attack before the headache develops? Anticipation of events can trigger migraine, particularly in children. Excitement is hard to avoid when someone is looking forward to a special occasion, but reducing other potential migraine triggers in the days leading up to the event may help. A long car journey can provoke several triggers: missed meals, neck ache, bright light from headlamps when driving at night, etc. Such triggers can be minimized by stopping for regular breaks and avoiding night driving. Acute treatments should not normally be used to prevent attacks but there is some evidence that the antisickness drug, domperidone can prevent migraine, when taken during the prodrome, before the headache has started. Sometimes, preventative drugs can be taken daily for a few days before regular anticipated attacks, such as when travelling or 'menstrual' migraine. Drugs should only be used in this way on a doctor's advice with caution against overuse. Stress-relieving strategies such as relaxation tapes, massage, yoga or breathing exercises can also help.

I am taking an increasing number of painkillers to relieve my migraine. Will they cause any long-term harm? Although painkillers are the mainstay of managing migraine, overuse can aggravate headache. Painkillers should not be taken regularly on more than a couple of days a week. Anyone taking them more often than this should see their doctor in order to find the cause of the frequent attacks. Painkillers taken in excess can cause liver and kidney problems.

I only used to get migraine once every couple of months but over the last year they've been getting more frequent. I now get them every day and nothing seems to help. Can I have something stronger to take? Daily headaches are not migraine and should not be treated as such. Further, taking drugs to control the symptoms does not treat the cause and may be exacerbating the condition. Stronger medication is not appropriate. Once sinister causes of headache have been excluded, daily painkillers should be stopped. This, in itself, may improve the headache and any residual headache can be diagnosed and treated with the correct treatment.

16

I know that I shouldn't take painkillers/ergots/triptans so often for my headaches but if I don't take them, I wouldn't be able to get to work, look after the kids, etc. Nothing else works. What can I do? The simple answer is that there is no substitute for stopping the acute treatments. Although the resultant headache may be severe in the short term, the long-term gain makes the effort worthwhile. Some patients feel more in control if they gradually reduce the drugs, taking reducing doses at the same time each day over several weeks. Additional drugs taken daily, such as amitriptyline, can be prescribed to aid the withdrawal process. Depending on the drug that has been misused, it may be possible for specific acute drugs to be taken for severe headache symptoms, although their use will be restricted during the withdrawal process. The first 2 weeks are usually the worse, with gradual improvement continuing up to 12 weeks later.

Hormones

I've started to get migraines regularly with my period. Is there anything wrong with my hormones? Most women are more likely to experience migraine at the time of their period. Menstruation acts as an additional trigger to all the usual triggers of missed meals, late nights, etc. In the same way that there is nothing wrong with late nights or missed meals, there is nothing wrong with the hormones. It is just that women with migraine are more sensitive to normal hormone changes.

I don't have migraine but my mother and grandmother did. I've heard that the contraceptive pill might trigger migraine, is this true? Migraine is a condition that starts in the teens and twenties, much the same time as many women start taking the pill. Therefore, it is not always easy to know if there is a true link between the two, or if it is just chance. Migraine is more commonly affected by the combined oral contraceptive pill than the progestogen-only pill. If severe headaches or migraine develop soon after starting the combined pill, it may be necessary to use alternative contraception.

16

I've been told that I can't take the pill because I get an aura with my migraine, but I can't risk getting pregnant. Is there any other effective contraceptive I can use? The combined pill is not suitable for women who have migraine with aura and should be discontinued immediately if any symptoms suggestive of reduced blood flow to the brain, including aura and other neurological symptoms, develop. This is because neurological symptoms, particularly when combined with the effect of synthetic oestrogen, are associated with an increased risk of stroke. Although this risk is very small, alternative effective contraception is available which does not increase the risk. Progestogen-only and non-hormonal contraceptive methods are suitable alternatives, some of which are more effective that the combined contraceptive pill.

I'm fine while I'm taking the pill but I often get attacks in the week I don't take it, when I get my period. Is there anything I can do to stop this happening? Levels of the synthetic oestrogen used in the pill, known as ethinyloestradiol, fall during the pill-free interval. Some women with migraine are sensitive to falling levels of oestrogen, which can trigger migraine. If effective migraine treatments are not sufficient to control symptoms, it is possible to take two or three packets of the pill consecutively. This reduces the number of pill-free intervals each year, and consequently the number of migraines, from 13 to seven or five.

My headaches got much worse when I started the pill, so much so that I've had to stop taking it. I stopped 6 weeks ago and they haven't improved. Why not? Studies show that it can take about 6 months for the effects of the pill to get completely out of the system. Most women improve after this time, although in a few, the pattern of attacks remains unchanged.

I've had bad headaches for years but now that I'm pregnant I've noticed that my vision goes funny and my hand feels weak for about 20 minutes before I get the headache. Am I having a stroke? In a few women, pregnancy seems to trigger attacks of migraine with aura. Studies show that typical symptoms of migraine aura are of no consequence to the mother, or the baby. However, visual symptoms can be indicative of serious conditions such as eclampsia. Therefore, it is important that any unusual symptom that develops during pregnancy is checked by a doctor.

16

I've hardly had any migraines since I've been pregnant. Will they come back when the baby is born? Migraine improves during pregnancy in over 70% of women, particularly during the second and third trimesters. The reasons for this improvement are unknown. Certainly, pregnancy marks a time of more stable hormone and blood sugar levels but women also look after themselves better, eating more regularly and taking more rest. After the baby is born, disrupted sleep and missed meals will certainly provoke attacks. The return of menstruation provides an additional trigger for many.

COMMON QUESTIONS AND ANSWERS

Will my baby be harmed if I have migraines when I'm pregnant? There is no evidence that migraine has any harmful effect on the baby.

What medication can I take for migraine while I'm pregnant? The only drug that can normally be recommended for use in pregnancy is paracetamol. It is important to discuss all medication with a doctor or pharmacist before they are taken. This includes vitamins and herbal treatments

I don't want to take any drugs while I'm pregnant. Is there any other advice you can give me to control bad attacks? Sleep is nature's way of treating migraine, so anything that helps promote sleep is useful. Resting in a quiet, darkened room, and using a cold or hot pad to ease the pain may help. Some patients have found relaxation techniques invaluable during pregnancy. In some areas, transcutaneous electrical nerve stimulation (TENS) machines are available on loan to help ease backache and early labour pains.

Can I breast-feed my baby while I'm taking medication for migraine? Always check with a pharmacist or doctor before taking any medication when breast-feeding, as certain drugs are secreted into breast milk and can affect the baby.

I've been told that a hysterectomy will cure my migraine. Is this true? The womb is only the end organ of the menstrual cycle. The master organ, implicated in both migraine and control of menstruation, is in the brain. Studies show that hysterectomy, particularly if the ovaries are also removed, is usually followed by worsening of migraine. However, this may be prevented by the use of hormone replacement therapy.

Will my migraines stop at the menopause? The menopause is a time of worsening migraine for many women. Fortunately, as hormones settle after the menopause, and hot flushes cease, so migraine become less frequent.

16

I've been told that hormone replacement therapy will cure my migraine. Is this true? Hormone replacement therapy can both aggravate and relieve migraine, depending on the type that is used. Since hormone fluctuations can trigger migraine, oral hormone replacement therapy, which provokes hormone fluctuations following each dose, may aggravate migraine. However, patches, gels and implants, all of which provide stable levels of hormones, may help migraine.

My migraines got worse around my menopause and I always believed they would get better when my periods stopped. I'm 62 now and they're as bad as ever. Why? Although hormone fluctuations do aggravate migraine, they are rarely the sole trigger. Certain triggers, particularly neck problems, may worsen with age. Not uncommonly, migraine gets better with the menopause but another headache develops. The doctor may need to check the diagnosis to ensure that the headache is treated correctly. Medication-misuse headache is another reason why headaches continue past the menopause.

Children

My son, aged 12 suffers from migraine. Will he grow out of it? Puberty is a difficult time for children, made harder if they also have headaches. In general, boys tend to have fewer problems with migraine than girls, although the growth spurt at puberty can be a difficult time.

My daughter, aged 12, suffers from migraine. Will she grow out of it? Unfortunately, girls tend to grow in to migraine. Most girls manage to cope with infrequent migraine during adolescence. The final years of reproduction mark the time of life when women have most problems with migraine, which usually improves after the menopause.

My daughter is about to take her GCSEs and gets frequent migraine. How can we prevent her having an attack on the day? Migraine usually occurs after, rather than during, stress. This means that although migraine may have disrupted studying for an exam, the child is usually unaffected on the day. However, if there is any cause for concern, if frequent migraines affect revision, or if several long exams are expected on consecutive days, a short course of β-blockers can be taken to prevent attacks. These should be tested well in advance of any exams to ensure that side-effects do not affect performance. Reduce other potential triggers by eating regularly, getting sufficient sleep (rather than burning the candle over the books), taking regular breaks and getting fresh air and exercise.

Should I let the school know that my child has migraine? It is always important to let the school know about any medical condition that may affect a child, particularly since the child could develop an attack while at school. Schools have differing policies on instigating treatment for chronic conditions. This should be discussed with all the relevant people concerned.

16

212

I'm not keen on my child becoming reliant on tablets to treat migraine. Is there anything else we can do? Studies show that the methods used by children to control migraine are the ones that they will rely on in later life. Simple analgesics for infrequent attacks should not be a cause for concern, provided they are effective. With regard to prevention, it is best to focus on non-drug methods where possible, reserving drugs for attacks that do not respond. Obviously, the best means of treatment is preventing attacks by identifying and avoiding triggers. But keep things in perspective. Parents can become over obsessive in trying to identify triggers, a situation that can end up disrupting the quality of life for the whole family. Other non-drug treatments are worth considering— biofeedback has been shown to be very effective in children.

Should I stop my child eating chocolate? Children often eat chocolate and are then too full to eat a proper meal. The real trigger is the missed meal, not the chocolate. There is no compelling evidence to suggest that, for the majority of children, giving up chocolate alone will prevent migraine.

Information

Where can I find out more information about migraine? Information about self-help groups is given in Appendix A.

How do I get to a migraine clinic? Addresses of a local migraine clinics can be found in Appendix A. Most clinics require a referral letter.

16

Useful Information

Professional organizations

International Headache Society (IHS)

Membership is open to all who are actively engaged or interested in clinical or research work in headache and related fields and have university or equivalent qualifications in a field applicable to the problem of headache, including medicine, surgery, psychiatry, medical or biological science, psychology, nursing or physical therapy, medical ethics or law. Membership includes subscription to *Cephalalgia*, an international headache journal.

Contact: Scandinavian University Press, PO Box 2959 Tøyen, N-0608 Oslo, Norway. Tel. +47 22 57 54 00; Fax: +47 22 57 53 53; Email: subscription@scup.no.

British Association for the Study of Headache (BASH)

Founded in 1993, this professional body is the national group of the International Headache Society. The objects of the Association are to relieve suffering from headache by the advancement of clinical management, research and education. Education is high on the list of priorities and programs of educational activity include GPs.

Contact: The Princess Margaret Migraine Clinic, Charing Cross Hospital, Fulham Palace Road, London W6 8RF. Tel. 0181 8461191; Fax: 0181 7417808.

Primary care

Migraine in Primary Care Advisors (MIPCA)

MIPCA Secretariat, PO Box 226, Richmond, Surrey TW9 1LU.

Lay organizations

Migraine Action Association

178a High Road, Byfleet, West Byfleet, Surrey KT14 7ED. Tel. 01932 352468;

Fax: 01932 351257; E-mail: info@migraine.org.uk; internet: www.migraine.org.uk.

The Migraine Trust

45 Great Ormond Street, London WC1N 3HZ, Tel. 0171 2782676; Fax: 0171 8314818; internet: www.migrainetrust.org.

Migraine clinics

Dedicated migraine clinics (adults and children)

The City of London Migraine Clinic

This registered medical charity accepts GP referrals from all over the UK at no charge to the referring doctor. Patients are requested to make a donation.

Contact: 22 Charterhouse Square, London EC1M 6DX. Tel. 0171 2513322.

The Princess Margaret Migraine Clinic

An NHS clinic. GP referral required.

Contact: Charing Cross Hospital, Fulham Palace Road, London W6 8RF. Tel. 0181 8461252.

Hospitals with headache/migraine clinics

All require GP referral.

Belfast: Royal Victoria Hospital, Grosvenor Road, Belfast BT12 6BA. Tel. 01232 240503, extension 3426.

Birmingham: The Queen Elizabeth Neurosciences Centre, Edgbaston, Birmingham B15 2TT. Tel. 0121 6272352. One session/week

Dublin: Neurology Department, Beaumont Hospital, Beaumont, Dublin 9. Tel. 0353 18093000.

Edinburgh: Western General Hospital, Edinburgh EH4 2XU. Tel. 0131 5372676. One session/week.

Guildford: Royal Surrey County Hospital, Egerton Road, Guildford, Surrey GU2 5XX. Tel. 01483 571122 extension 4849. One session/week.

Hull: Department of Neurology, Hull Royal Infirmary, Anlaby Road, Hull HU3 2JZ. Tel. 01482 675591. Three sessions/week.

Ipswich: Department of Clinical Neurology, The Ipswich Hospital NHS Trust, Heath Road, Ipswich IP4 5PD. Tel. 01473 703188. Three sessions/week.

Leicester: Department of Neurology, Leicester Royal Infirmary, Leicester LE1 5WW. Tel. 0116 2585380. One to two sessions/week.

London: The Migraine Research Clinic, Hammersmith Hospital, Du Cane Road, London W12 0HS. Tel. 0181 3838999 (Research only).

London: King's College Hospital, Denmark Hill, London SE5. Tel. 0171 3465357. Two sessions/week.

London: The National Hospital, Queen Square, London WC1N 3ZG. Tel. 0171 8373611 extension 8749. One to two sessions/week.

London: The Royal London Hospital, Whitechapel, London E1 1BB. Tel. 0171 3777472. Two sessions/month.

Manchester: Department of Neurology, Manchester Royal Infirmary, Oxford Road, Manchester M13 9WL. Tel. 0161 2764149. One session/week.

Manchester: Department of Neurology, Withington Hospital, West Didsbury, Manchester M20 2LR. Tel. 0161 2913489. One session/week.

Oxford: Department of Neurology, The Radcliffe Infirmary, Woodstock Road, Oxford OX2 6HE. Tel. 01865 224923. Two sessions/week.

Preston: Royal Preston Hospital, Sharoe Green, Preston, Lancs PR2 4HT. Tel. 01772 710423. One session/week.

Sheffield: Department of Neurology, Royal Hallamshire Hospital, Glossop Road, Sheffield S10 2JF. Tel. 0114 2711900. One session/week.

Sunderland: Department of Neurology, Sunderland Royal Hospital, Kayll Road, Sunderland, Tyne and Wear SR4 7TP. Tel. 0191 5656256. One session/week.

Wakefield: Pinderfields General Hospital, Aberford Road, Wakefield WF1 4DG. Tel. 01924 212359. One session/week.

York: Department of Neurosciences, York District Hospital, Wigginton Road, York YO3 7HE. Tel. 01904 454161. One session/week.

Neurology clinics with an interest in headache

Note: all patients with headache can be referred to neurology outpatient departments of the local hospitals. The following hospitals have doctors with a special interest in headache.

Basildon: Department of Neurology, Nether Mayne, Basildon, Essex SS16 5NL. Tel. 01268 593428.

Colchester: Neurocare Unit, Colchester General Hospital, Colchester CO4 5JL. Tel. 01206 832526.

Newcastle upon Tyne: Department of Neurology, Royal Victoria Infirmary, Queen Victoria Road, Newcastle upon Tyne NE1 4LP. Tel. 0191 2822949.

Nottingham: Department of Neurology, University Hospital, Queen's Medical Centre, Nottingham NG7 2UH. Tel. 01159 249924.

Portsmouth: Department of Neurology, St Mary's Hospital, Milton Road, Portsmouth PO3 8LD. Tel. 01705 286000 extension 3820.

Romford: Essex Neurosciences Unit, Oldchurch Hospital, Romford, Essex RM7 0BE. Tel. 01708 708223.

A

Southampton: Wessex Neurological Centre, Southampton General Hospital, Tremona Road, Southampton SO16 6YD. Tel. 01703 777222.

Paediatric clinics

Aberdeen: Paediatric Department, Stirling Royal Infirmary, Stirling, Scotland. Tel. 01786 434000. One session/week.
Hartlepool: Paediatric Department, General Hospital, Holdforth Road, Hartlepool TS24 9AX. Tel. 01429 522802. One session/week.
Stirling: Royal Aberdeen Children's Hospital, Cornhill Road, Aberdeen. Tel. 01224 681818 extension 53564. Two sessions/month.

Videos for doctors

A Three Minute Migraine History. Useful advice on eliciting the salient diagnostic points.

A Three Minute Neurological Examination for use in Recurrent Headaches. This video provides useful information on how to cover the essentials of a neurological examination in headache patients.

Both can be obtained from: Zeneca Pharma, King's Court, Water Lane, Wilmslow, Cheshire SK9 5A.

Assessment of management

Migraine review

A tool designed to help GPs regularly review management of their migraine patients by supporting clinical outcomes, facilitating appropriate prescribing and aiding the development of practice standards.

For further information contact: GlaxoWellcome Customer Service. Tel. 0800 221441; Fax: 0181 9904328.

Oxygen for cluster headache

A

BOC Medical Gases (contact local branch)

BOC supply a regulator and face mask which will deliver the necessary 6–9 litres oxygen per minute at a high flow rate.
Multiflow regulator code 888842—available only from BOC cost approx £100 but may be possible to rent.
Face mask code 888845—available on prescription.
Standard 1360-litre cylinder 137 bar—available on prescription.

Further Reading

Blau JN (ed). *Migraine: Clinical, Therapeutic, Conceptual and Research Aspects.* Cambridge, Chapman and Hall Medical, 1987.

Managing migraine. *Drugs Ther Bull* 1998; 36: 41–44.

Lance JW. *Mechanisms and Management of Headache,* 5th edn. Oxford, Butterworth Heinemann, 1993.

Mathew NT (ed). Advances in headache. *Neurol Clin* 1997; 15: 1–238.

Olesen J, Tfelt-Hansen P, Welch KMA (eds). *The Headaches.* New York, Raven Press, 1993.

Silberstein SD, Lipton RB, Goadsby PJ. *Headache in Clinical Practice.* Oxford, ISIS Medical Media, 1998.

Sjaastad O. Cluster headache syndrome. *Major Problems in Neurology,* Vol. 23. London, WB Saunders Company, 1992.

Tate P. *The Doctor's Communication Handbook.* Oxford, Radcliffe Medical Press, 1994.

Journals

Cephalalgia (Journal of the International Headache Society), Scandinavian University Press, PO Box 2959 Tøyen, N-0608 Oslo, Norway. Tel. +47 22 57 54 00; Fax: +47 22 57 53 53; E-mail: subscription@scup.no.

Headache (Journal of the American Association for the Study of Headache), 19 Mantua Road, Mt Royal, New Jersey 08061, USA. Tel. +1609 4230043; Fax: +1609 4230082; E-mail: aashhq@aash.smarthub.com; internet: WWW: http://www.aash.org.

Books for patients

Blau JN. *Understanding Headaches and Migraine.* Which Consumer Guides, 1991. ISBN 0340518626. Price £8.95.

Wilkinson M & MacGregor A. *Understanding Migraine and Other Headaches.* Family Doctor Publications, 1995. ISBN 1898205043. Price £2.49.

B

Auditing Migraine

Why audit?

- Because audit activity is expected.
- It can lead to improved patient care.
- It can be thought provoking, educational and interesting.

Why migraine?

- It is very common, but not all patients consult, so the audit should not take too long.
- Migraine can be associated with high morbidity with time lost from work and leisure.
- Previous studies have shown that there is potential for improvement in the diagnosis and management of migraine.
- Simple tools can aid diagnosis of migraine in primary care.
- Assessment of particular subgroups can lead to development of more optimal care, for example 'triptan' users (simple management strategies can be as effective for some patients), combined oral contraceptive users, hormone replacement therapy users, elderly patients (is it still migraine?), children, daily headaches (is it medication misuse ± migraine?)
- Any improvement is often manageable without an excessive time commitment.
- It will benefit patients.
- It may benefit communication with secondary care.

Strategy

Whilst it is a good idea for one member of the Practice to promote the audit, it is important that all GPs and staff become involved. Involvement of all members of the team in this discussion may generate enthusiasm and commitment to the project.

Is it migraine?

How many different types of headaches does the patient have? Ask the following questions for each headache.

- How often are the headaches? Migraine headaches are episodic with complete freedom from symptoms between attacks. Daily headaches are not migraine although migraine can arise on a background of daily headache.
- How long do the headaches last? Migraine typically lasts for part to 1 day, but may last from 4 h to 3 days.
- Are there any warning signs of an impending attack? Migraine can be preceded by subtle 'prodromal' changes in mood or behaviour including depression, extreme lethargy, elation, and food cravings which occur several hours, or even the day, before the onset of headache. Thirty per cent of attacks are preceded by a neurological aura, typically of bright zigzags (fortification spectra) spreading across the visual field, lasting 20–60 min before the onset of headache. It usually resolves as the headache develops.
- Is there nausea and/or vomiting? Migraine is typically accompanied with nausea and/or vomiting.
- Is there photophobia or phonophobia?
- Is the headache throbbing?
- Is the headache one-sided? Seventy per cent are unilateral but 30% are bilateral.

Step 1: preparing for the audit

Arrange a meeting of all the partners. Consider inviting practice nurses and office staff, especially if they are going to do some of the work collecting information.

The purpose of the meeting is to consider what your practice thinks of the standards of care for your patients with migraine should be.

Possible discussion points may include some of the following.
- What are the aims of treatment? Should patients be completely free of migraine? How much should treatment be should be decided jointly with the patient?
- Which antimigraine drugs would you consider to be first-line acute treatments?
- When should patients be offered prophylactic therapy, which drug, and for how long?
- Which patients with migraine can still use the combined oral contraceptive pill?
- How often should patients with migraine be seen by their GP?
- Which patients suspected of having migraine should be referred to a consultant?
- Should such patients be regularly followed up by a hospital consultant?
- What information should be recorded in the notes? Should recording the number of migraines per month in the last 3 months be an aim?

C

• What information should patients with migraine be given and who should give it? For example, identification and avoidance of trigger factors, information to keep on diary cards.

Someone needs to record what the practice consensus is on these discussion points, then—hey presto! You have your practice's own standards of care for your patients with migraine.

Step 2: collecting the information

A member of staff (this could be a GP, a receptionist, practice nurse or secretary) should scrutinize the repeat prescriptions for 3 months, and keep a list of patients who are taking antimigraine drugs, or combinations of analgesics with antiemetics. An average group practice would expect to see 80 new presentations of migraine per year and 20 repeat sufferers. It is worth noting that this represents only a small proportion of the estimated prevalence of migraine in the community, estimated to be around 12%.

Alternative methods might be to use your computer. Remember some GPs may issue repeat prescriptions on home visits, and some patients may get their drugs from hospital. If you can remember who these patients are, that is fine, if not, it does not matter too much.

This should identify all the patients who have migraine in the practice except:
• those who do not take prescribed medication, i.e. they use over-the-counter treatments which may or may not be recommended by the doctor;
• those who are taking non-specific analgesics, like paracetamol, for migraine—these could be identified by assessing all patients using prescription analgesics but would increase the workload;
• those who have a history of migraine but are no longer treated.

Obtain notes for all identified patients. (Receptionist?)

Scrutinize notes to see why these patients are taking antimigraine drugs. (Doctor, practice nurse, registrar?)

Discard patients who do not have a history of headache or migraine. Some will be taking acute treatments for other pain, and prophylaxis for hypertension, or depression. Note: this may be quite a few and it may be difficult to decide clearly.

Collect information required to complete the enclosed grids (see Table A1, p. 225). (Doctor/Practice nurse/nurse practitioner?) The following pieces of information as outlined on the next pages may be useful, but you will possibly be interested in other topics. Remember that each additional item searched for increases the time taken. This job is the most time consuming. Depending on the state of your records, allow 10 min per set of notes.

C

Suggested areas of information to collect

- Practice list size?
- Number of patients identified with migraine?

For each patient

- Age?
- Sex?
- Has a diagnosis of headache/migraine been recorded?
- Can you be sure it is migraine? (See checklist.)
- Number of patients with daily headaches instead, or in addition to, migraine?
- What reasons for consulting did each patient give, for example increased frequency, severity, new symptoms, pressure from family/work?
- Acute and/or prophylaxis?
- Which drug/s each patient is taking? (Use enclosed list and codes.)
- Does the repeat prescription match the notes?
- When was each patient last seen for any reason?
- When was each patient last seen about their migraine?
- Frequency of consultations for headache/migraine in the last 2 years? (If recorded.)
- Which patients have been referred to a hospital consultant about the migraine and why?
- Has written information about migraine and its management been provided, and recorded in the notes?
Your additions if required.

Step 3: making sense of the information

How you approach this section will very much depend on what you decide and 'Step 1: preparing for the audit', where you will have decided your areas of priority.

The following suggestions may help to clarify your thoughts for assessing the data, but feel free to add any of your identified areas:

- How many patients in each age band: 0–10, 11–20, 21–30, etc.
- How many males/females—percentage.
- Reason for consulting.
- Percentage of each antimigraine drug (or standard combination) used against a total of all antimigraine drugs (acute and prophylactic).
- Patient last seen, any reason—last month, 1–3 months, 4–6 months, 7–12 months, 12+ months.
- Patient last seen for migraine—categories as previous question.
- Frequency of consultations in the last 2 years—weekly, monthly, every few months, less often.

C

- How many patients have been referred to a hospital consultant for migraine—percentage of total identified in the practice.
- Reasons given for the referral.
- A record of information on migraine given—percentage yes/no.

Step 4: discussing what you have discovered

The practice team needs to re-convene to discuss the findings. It helps if someone records the Practice's conclusions.

- Present results.
- Discuss the implications.
- Plan the future management of patients with migraine—you may want to make some changes.
- Decide on a time for the next audit—it is a good idea to repeat the exercise to see if you have improved patient care.
- The audit process may raise important unanswered questions about certain patients. These may require contact with an hospital consultant, other Primary Health Care Team members or social services.

Reason(s) for patient consulting

Code	Reason stated
1	Increased frequency of attacks.
2	Increased severity of attacks.
3	Onset of new symptoms.
4	Fear of underlying pathology.
5	Treatment failure.
6	Pressure from friends/family.
7	Pressure from employer.
8	Other reason.

Reason(s) for referral to specialist

Code	Reason stated
9	Diagnostic concerns.
10	Treatment failure.
11	Investigation of suspected pathology.
12	Patient request.

Drug list

Code	Drug name
1	Analgesics only (if identified)—over-the-counter = 1A, prescription-only medicine = 1B.
2	Migraleve.

Table A1

Name of practice: _____   Practice list size: _____

Initials of patient: _____

Actual age (enter exact age)			
Sex (enter M or F)			
Which acute drugs (enter exact code no. or NR)			
Which prophylactic drugs (enter exact code no. or NR)			
Prescription matches notes (enter Y, N, or NR)			
Patient last seen, any reason (enter date by month/year, or NR)			
Patient last seen, migraine (enter date by month/year, or NR)			
Frequency of consultations in the last 2 years for migraine (enter frequency or NR)			
Referral to hospital consultant for migraine (enter Y, N, or NR)			
Reasons given for the referral (record reason, or NR)			
Information on migraine given (enter Y, N, or NR)			

C

3	Midrid.
4	Migravess.
5	Paramax.
6	Domperamol.
7	Tolfenamic acid (Clotam).
8	Other combination of analgesic/antiemetic.
9	Ergotamine (any form, e.g. Migril, Cafergot, Lingraine, Medihaler).
10	Sumatriptan (Imigran).
11	Naratriptan (Naramig).
12	Zolmitriptan (Zomig).
20	β-blocker (e.g. propranolol).
21	Tricyclic antidepressant (e.g. amitriptyline).
22	Selective serotonin re-uptake inhibitor SSRI (e.g. fluoxetine).
23	Pizotifen (Sanomigran).
24	Sodium valproate (Epilim).
25	Methysergide (Deseril).
26	Other prophylactic.

Audit credit

This audit was prepared with help from Dr Bill Hall, GP, Settle, North Yorkshire and Brian Chappell, NEUROEDUCATION. Other audits based on the same methodology are available from NEUROEDUCATION, PO Box 17, Golcar, Huddersfield, HD7 4YX. They are free and cover epilepsy, multiple sclerosis and Parkinson's disease.

C

The City of London Migraine Clinic

The City of London Migraine Clinic was founded, in its present guise, as a registered medical charity in 1980 by Dr Nat Blau and Dr Marcia Wilkinson, both of whom are consultant neurologists with a particular interest in migraine.

Its initial aims were to provide a 'walk-in' service for patients during acute migraine attacks, as well as acting as a research centre into the causes and better treatment of migraine. Research undertaken on patients led to the identification of effective acute therapy with aspirin and metoclopramide, a combination that is now offered as a standard line of management. Although we still offer emergency treatment, most of our patients are now referred by their GPs for advice on diagnosis and management.

The Clinic offers a unique service, being free to both patient and the referring GP—hence doctors can see patients from all over the UK. Unlike a busy NHS setting, the Clinic offers an unhurried thorough consultation carried out in a quiet 18th century building. There is a clear demand for the continuance of the service as increasing numbers of patients are being referred.

Research into the causes and better management of migraine and other headaches continues. New drugs and non-drug treatments for migraine are tested at the clinic in scientifically controlled clinical trials. The Clinic is recognized as an international centre of high repute, with doctors visiting from all over the world to gain further experience of headache management.

Doctors and other healthcare professionals with an interest in headache are encouraged to visit the clinic. Visits can be arranged by contacting:

The City of London Migraine Clinic
22 Charterhouse Square
London EC1M 6DX
Tel. 0171 2513322
Fax: 0171 4902183

D

IHS and WHO Criteria

Adapted from: Headache Classification Committee of the International Headache Society. Classification and Diagnostic Criteria for Headache Disorders, Cranial Neuralgias and Facial Pain. *Cephalalgia* 1988; 8 (Suppl. 7): 1–96.

See also: *ICD-10 Guide for Headaches*. WHO guide to the classification, diagnosis and assessment of headaches in accordance with the Tenth Revision of the International Classification of Diseases and Related Health Problems and its Application to Neurology.

Note: IHS codes given first followed by WHO codes in parentheses.

Primary headaches

Code 1 (G43): migraine

Code 1.1 (G43.0): migraine without aura (common migraine)

Description: Idiopathic, recurring headache disorder manifesting in attacks lasting 4–72 h. Typical characteristics of headache are unilateral location, pulsating quality, moderate or severe intensity, aggravation by routine physical activity, and association with nausea, photo- and phonophobia.

Diagnostic criteria:
A At least five attacks fulfilling B–D.
B Headache attacks, lasting 4–72 h (untreated or unsuccessfully treated).
C Headache has at least two of the following characteristics:
    1 unilateral location;
    2 pulsating quality;
    3 moderate or severe intensity (inhibits or prohibits daily activities);
    4 aggravation by walking stairs or similar routine activity.
D During headache at least one of the following:
    1 nausea and/or vomiting;
    2 photophobia and phonophobia.

Code 1.2 (G43.1): migraine with aura (classical migraine)

Description: Idiopathic, recurring disorder manifesting with attacks of neurological symptoms unequivocally localizable to cerebral cortex or

E

brainstem, usually gradually developed over 5–20 min and usually lasting less than 60 min. Headache, nausea and/or photophobia usually follow neurological aura symptoms directly or after a free interval of less than 1 h. The headache usually lasts 4–72 h, but may be completely absent.

Diagnostic criteria:

A At least two attacks fulfilling B.

B At least three of the following four characteristics.
1   One or more fully reversible aura symptoms indicating focal cerebral cortical and/or brainstem dysfunction.
2   At least one aura symptom develops gradually over more than 4 min or two or more symptoms occur in succession.
3   No aura symptom lasts more than 60 min. If more than one aura symptom is present, accepted duration is proportionally increased.
4   Headache follows aura with a free interval of less than 60 min, but may begin before or simultaneously with the aura.

Code 1.2.1 (G43.10): migraine with typical aura

A Fulfills criteria for 1.2 including all four criteria under B.

B One or more aura symptoms of the following types:
1   homonymous visual disturbance;
2   unilateral paraesthesias and/or numbness;
3   unilateral weakness;
4   aphasia or unclassifiable speech difficulty.

Code 1.2.2 (G43.11): migraine with prolonged aura

Code 1.2.3 (G43.1x5): familial hemiplegic migraine

Code 1.2.4 (G43.1x3): basilar migraine

Code 1.2.5 (G43.1x4): migraine aura without headache

Code 1.2.6 (G43.12): migraine with acute-onset aura

Code 1.3 (G43.80): ophthalmoplegic migraine

Code 1.4 (G43.81): retinal migraine

Code 1.5 (G43.82): childhood periodic syndromes that may be precursors to or associated with migraine

Code 1.6 (G43.3): complications of migraine

E

Code 1.7 (G43.9): migrainous disorder not fulfilling above criteria

Code 2 (G44.2): tension-type headache

Code 3 (G44.0): cluster headache and chronic paroxysmal hemicrania

Code 4 (G44.80): miscellaneous headaches unassociated with structural lesion

Secondary headaches

Code 5 (G44.3): headache associated with head trauma

Code 6 (G44.81): headache associated with vascular disorders

Code 7 (G44.82): headache associated with non-vascular intracranial disorder

Code 8 (G44.4 and G44.83): headache associated with substances or their withdrawal

Code 9 (G44.881): headache associated with non-cephalic infection

Code 10 (G44.882): headache associated with metabolic disorder

Code 11 (G44.84 and G44.85): headache or facial pain associated with disorder of cranium, neck, eyes, nose sinuses, teeth, mouth or other facial or cranial structures

Code 12 (G44.847 and G44.848): cranial neuralgias, nerve trunk pain and deafferation pain

Code 13 (R51): headache not classifiable

E

Index

DATE DUE

OCT 3 0 2001			
OCT 1 0 2002 ILL			
NOV 0 4 2002			
GAYLORD			PRINTED IN U.S.A.